STRENGTH TRAINING

FOR MEN AND WOMEN OVER 50 RECLAIM YOUR
HEALTH & FITNESS LOSE FAT, GET TONED & BUILD
MUSCLE

ALICIA DIAZ

LEE DAVIDSON

OTHER TITLES IN THE
LIFE AFTER 50 SERIES

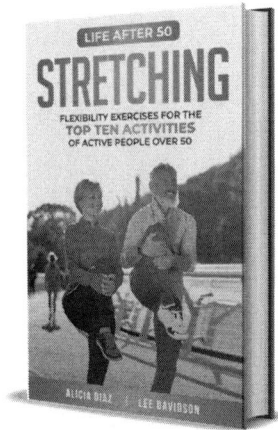

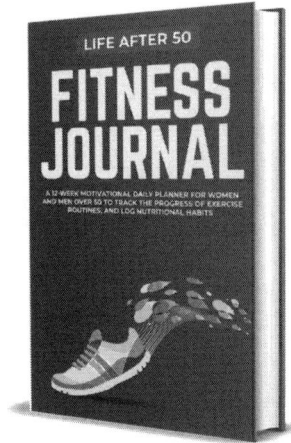

For more information
on these titles, visit:
healthylifeafter50.com
or...

SCAN ME

TABLE OF CONTENTS

Just For You!

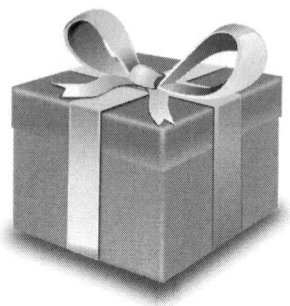

A FREE GIFT TO OUR READERS

CLAIM YOUR GIFT AT:
healthylifeafter50.com
...or

SCAN ME

INTRODUCTION

For the past couple of years we've been on a mission (and yes, sometimes it seems more like mission impossible). Many 50+ers seem to have slipped into some kind of "old-age trance." While in that trance, they accept that when they break through the border of 50, they're **destined** to be plagued with aches, pains, and inflexibility. They **accept** it and seemingly make room for these discomforts in their lives. This has to change.

Sadly, many 50+ers believe that being fit, flexible, and agile is only for **some** people. Somehow, they think that only a **lucky few** get to head into 50 and even 60, still able to touch their toes, reach for something or head out for a run or round of golf. The reality is harsh; we get that. You've spent the majority of your life scrambling after children and chasing careers, and now that you've hit fifty and life is slowing down, you're left with that "Woah, what happened?" feeling.

Here come the aches and pains because, well, you haven't been moving as much as you used to when you were twenty. You undoubtedly spent Saturdays in your 30's and 40's trying to catch up on laundry (which may seem like an Olympic event, but it's not) and stressing over your children's educations. You spent more time on the couch (trying not to assume the fetal position) on Sundays than anywhere near a sporting facility, and perhaps you don't even own a pair of running shoes or a gym bag by this stage. Your life got busy, but not in an active way. What a conundrum!

It all makes sense that bending, touching your toes, or even doing a few squats (not even for exercise – merely to pick something up) take it out of you. Your body resists with all its might. It strikes back with aches and pains and if it has the strength to muster it, strains too. And you translate all of this bodily reaction to mean "I don't *want* to exercise or move" or "I *can't* exercise or move" when in reality, the body is saying something else entirely. Don't worry; we don't blame you for not understanding. Are you curious what the *real* message is? Here goes:

> *"I need to get stronger!"*

And now that you know what that message is, what are you going to do about it? Of course, the first step is reading this book. And without giving you too much of a spoiler alert, we'd like to explain *why* you should read it. First and foremost, it's about knowledge. Knowing what you're in for in the 50+ club will help you find methods and strategies of not just coping but thriving. You need to thrive because as you get older, your muscles and joints weaken. This isn't a foregone conclusion, by the way. Unfortunately, this is where people go wrong. You read something like "muscles and joints weaken as you age," and you accept it when in reality, the truth is that muscles and joints *that aren't worked out and maintained* weaken as you age.

Suppose you're willing to do the maintenance on your body just as religiously as you do your vehicle or household maintenance. In that case, you may discover (and we mean you *will*) that your muscles, joints, and bones hold out pretty well. Another thing that changes as you age is the range of movement, overall strength, and blood circulation. Hey, you're getting older, so it's entirely acceptable that things slow down a little. That's okay, but how much are you willing to let things slow down?

Are you the type of person willing to spend your sixties glued to a sofa because everything seems like too much physical effort? Or are you the spry sixty-something-year-old visiting friends, playing golf, going on long walks (maybe even jogs), and carrying your groceries? Well, if you want to be the latter, your fifties is the perfect time to start making lifestyle changes that support that spry sixty-something ideal. What if we told you that learning to strengthen your muscles, joints, and bones is the answer? You merely have to learn to incorporate more dedicated techniques into your daily life, and all this talk of aches and pains would be a distant memory. That's why you have to read this book! Not just to learn about **why** your body changes but also to learn how to mitigate changes and stay younger, fitter, and stronger for longer. At this particular point, you're probably wondering who we are and why you should be taking our advice on strength training or anything else 50+ fitness-related at all. So here's what you need to know.

Our names are Alicia Diaz and Lee Davidson, and we're just like you. By that, we mean that we've already had our big 5-0 birthday celebrations, and we're well on our way to the next decade. We're both physically active at this point in our lives, and not a day goes by that we don't train. We spend much of our time hiking and running, playing tennis and golf, and we don't just do this as "sport" – these are things we do for recreation and socializing. Your daily to-do-list gets a little shorter after 50, and keeping fit and active has been our go-to. But, it hasn't always been this way. Well, let's rephrase that. We used to be extremely fit and active in our twenties. In fact, we lived for sporting activities.

> *"But then we did what most couples do and had kids".*

Having kids is a whirlwind adventure on its own, and if you have any, you will know just how challenging (or impossible) it is to keep up with your favorite sports and hobbies when those bundles of joy come along. Your gym kit becomes a comfy pair of pajamas, Saturday morning runs transition into baby playdates, and Sundays on the golf course are thwarted by the constant need to keep mini-humans alive.

Athletics and anything remotely sports and fitness-related takes a back seat. There may be a gym class or a walk that happens here and there, but it's not like it used to be. Soon, before you know it, you're well into your forties, and your feet don't even recognize running shoes anymore.

You probably know where this story is going. We both hit our fifties and bid our children a fond farewell as they flew out of the nest to live their own exciting lives. And there we were, just us and a quiet and empty nest. The next phase of life had come for us. *Empty nesters!* And this is where most people stop and fall into that trance we mentioned earlier. People will just assume their role as "old people" and embrace it. Here's a reality check: Life does not stop when your kids leave home and you head into your fifties. Instead, your life picks up where you left off in your twenties – active/fitness-wise, that is. And it was the arrival of our three beautiful grandchildren that delivered us this stark reality. We genuinely didn't have the time or option of slowing down and becoming weak, tired, and frail. Instead, we had three little faces staring up at us and wanting us to play, carry, run, and get involved.

Cue the aches, pains, and muscular strains - what a wake-up call! It was around this time that we deciphered the message from our bodies. We needed to strengthen and maintain ourselves (our bodies). We've never really looked back. While we currently do strength training and play plenty of sports and activities, stretching and strength training was where we started - after years of inactivity. And that's where we believe you should start too. In the last ten years, we have taken our fitness to the next level, and because of our active involvement in the community, we have had many 50+ers approach us and ask what our secret is. The thing is, we're agile, flexible, fit, strong, and active, and we didn't get this way through a secret or magic potion. Strength training is freely available to anyone who is able and wants to try it.

We've worked alongside nutritionists and physiotherapists to learn everything required about combining strength training and nutrition for the best possible results in the 50+ years. We've also done a lot of traveling and group talks to get the word out there that there's power in strength training at 50+, and this is something we genuinely believe. This brings us to writing this book. It's just another way of reaching out to our people, the community of 50+ers who want to live a more comfortable life. So, if you're a 50+er who is ready and willing to take the plunge and seize control of your life, then you're ready to read this book. You're ready to join us in waking yourself and others up from that "old-age" trance! There's only one thing left to do – turn the page to chapter one: *Staying Strong After 50.*

Alica Diaz & Lee Davidson

STAYING STRONG AFTER 50

The very first morning you wake up after you've just turned 50, you open your eyes and feel the dawn of a new era descend on you. There's an element of excitement as you enter a phase of fewer responsibilities and more freedom. But then, as you swing your legs out of bed and get ready to start the day, you wonder, "what now?" What do *other* people do when they don't have kids to fuss over and keep alive? And that's the clincher, isn't it? If you were, say, 30 years younger, you might have thrown yourself out of bed, dragged your running shoes on, and hit the sidewalk for some fresh air and a bit of a workout, but it's been so long since you've done that, that it seems almost unnatural.

DESIGNED FOR LIFELONG MOVEMENT

You were born to move

Before you head out to buy a set of knitting needles and a ball of wool (or, for the guys, a wood carving set), we'd like to share a secret with you; you were born to move. In a study (https://pubmed.ncbi.nlm.nih.gov/ 27723159) of the Hadza people (they're from Tanzania, by the way), researchers found that the Hadza people have excellent cardiovascular health. In short, the study found that humans are not well suited to the screen-focused and inactive lifestyles that have sadly become the norm in western society. Most people struggle to hit the recommended 150 minutes per week of moderate cardiovascular exercise for heart health. That said, the Hadza people (of all ages and regardless of season) participate in more than two hours of moderate to high-intensity exercise per day. This seems to be why they enjoy such exemplary heart heath. From this, we can deduce that we are designed to move a *lot* more than we do. But now, we have adapted to our sedentary lifestyle and barely move at all. Cue the heart conditions. Of course, this isn't just about old age – humans as a whole are primed from a young age (thanks to society) to spend more time sitting down behind a screen than they do moving around or exercising outside. It's just the way it is. So now you know, you're designed to move, but you haven't been moving for quite some time. What now? Just because you've got out of the habit of moving, flexing, and stretching at a higher speed than walking pace, it doesn't mean you're doomed to be achy, stiff, and inflexible forever. It simply means you have to get **back into** the habit.

Being designed for movement means that you can and will become flexible and fit again if you're willing to be consistent about it. If you played sports or indulged in exercise in your youth, you might remember that it didn't come naturally then either. You had to work on your fitness, flexibility, and skill – and it's the same now that you're older. Your muscles may have forgotten what it feels like to move and stretch the way they used to, but if you put in a little bit of work every day or even every week, you will notice how quickly they (your muscles, that is) are willing to learn new things and even excel at them.

THE DOWNSIDES OF AGING

While we are designed for movement, it's good to be aware of the result of aging. Applying the Ostrich method and simply avoiding the uncomfortable truth about aging won't help you. We have found that being aware of the "side effects" of aging and applying a few home remedies (in the form of exercise and strength training) has served us very well in the past few years. And we have seen it work for others too.

In the spirit of full disclosure, aging doesn't discriminate – it comes for us all. And unfortunately, it's one of those visitors that brings a few unwelcome guests with it. We're talking about lack of flexibility, decreased energy, reduced strength, increased risk of injury, stiffness, aches and pains, a sluggish metabolism, and a lack of confidence/self-esteem to boot. Of course, nobody welcomes these guests, but still, they come. Before you get too glum about the effects of aging, there's another secret we would like to share with you.

> *"Regular strength training and moderate exercise can send all those unwelcome old-age guests packing!"*

Let's briefly look at each of the most common downsides of aging that you may be experiencing right now. Unfortunately, these are often the very things that hold 50+ers back from rejoining the sport and fitness world. But, in reality, exercise can help you to overcome these issues.

Declining Muscle Mass

One of the biggest unwelcome visitors of old age is declining muscle mass. It doesn't matter if you're male or female; the idea of dwindling muscles is upsetting. That said, muscle mass affects men a little more than it affects women. According to Harvard Medical School (https://www.health.harvard.edu/staying-healthy/preserve-your-muscle-mass), when you reach 30, your muscles go into decline. In fact, you can lose as much as 3 to 5% of your muscle mass per decade. And when muscle mass declines, other things start to go awry too. For starters, you're at a greater risk of fracturing hip bones, collarbones, legs, arms, and wrists when falling. This is thanks to increased weakness and declining mobility – both nasty side effects of declining muscle mass.Declining muscle mass is the result of a combination of things happening to and in your body. Firstly, you're less active when you get older (or you have gradually become less active over the years), and then you're also going through hormonal changes as your body ages. No one wants to think about their muscles melting away; if anything, we would prefer that our fat would melt away! While declining muscle mass is a fact of life in old age, you can increase your muscle mass and maintain it by introducing strength training and a protein-rich diet to your daily/weekly routine.

Flexibility Declines

Do you remember being able to sit cross-legged on the floor and then quickly stand up without crawling around to a nearby furniture item for help or clinging to someone else to get you back up on your feet? Okay, perhaps it's not that dramatic yet, but it can become that bad if you neglect your physical fitness for much longer. Inactivity and lack of stretching are the top reasons for becoming inflexible, and the good news is that it's not only a problem that plagues older people (yay!). People in their 30s living a sedentary life will struggle to stretch, bend, or even touch their toes if they have never done a stitch of exercise, so there's no reason to feel alone in this.

As you age, your body starts to lose small amounts of flexibility along the way steadily. Some reasons for this include loss of water in the tissues and spine (a natural part of aging), stiff joints, and loss of muscle elasticity. When you're not feeling very flexible, you may find yourself decreasing your physical activities because you feel like you "can't do it." You may sit out on the sidelines while friends play a friendly round of tennis or even avoid climbing the stairs unless you have to (we've all been there – elevators are such a blessing!). Unfortunately, this will only lead to a bigger problem. The human body is all about "use it or lose it." If you don't stretch and use your muscles often, those types of movements will be considered unnecessary, and your body forgets all about them. Before you know it, your muscles feel weak and stiff at the mere thought of specific movements or exercises.

One day when your kids send you a package for your birthday, and the shipping company dumps it on your doorstep, you may experience all manner of aches, pains, and strains, just from bending down and picking it up. And in real-life terms, you may find yourself saying, "no, grandma can't pick you up today" or "sorry, grandpa can't run up the stairs with you" to your grandchildren a little more often than you'd like to.

Inflexibility can also lead to other uncomfortable issues over and above aches, pains, and disappointing your grandkids. These include walking slowly (or shuffling), only being able to take short steps/strides, increased fall risk (you're a little more unstable when the muscles are weak), and pesky back pain.

This all seems a little bleak, but the good news (again) is that you can improve and maintain a healthy level of flexibility with regular strength training and stretching. Of course, strength training isn't a magic bullet. A certain level of flexibility loss with age is unavoidable, but you can slow down the effects with the right approach and ensure you're still striding and skipping along well past the point of 50!

Studies have proven that strength training can be pretty miraculous when it comes to building muscle mass and increasing flexibility. For instance, building strength in the front hip muscles will promote steady walking speed and keep those strides lengthy and confident. You will also experience improved balance thanks to those stronger muscles pulling you firmly onto your feet. Thank goodness, right?

Achy Joints & Arthritis

Most people accept joint pain and arthritis as some sort of right of passage when aging, but the truth is that making healthy changes early on can help you thwart the severity of this part of the aging process. Rheumatologists may even tell you that while joint pains are more common in older folk, they are not guaranteed facts of life. You don't *have* to be that sore and achy. You can live a relatively pain-free life even after 50! Let's talk about the *types* of arthritis, as this can help you understand how making changes can stave off those aches and pains waiting to settle into your joints.

The first type we would like to focus on is OA, otherwise known as ***Osteoarthritis***. This is first up on the list because it is the most common type of arthritis. It results from wear and tear, meaning you have repeated the same movement over and over. Now your joints are getting a bit of revenge. This can also happen if you start using joints too soon after an injury. In this type of arthritis, the cartilage cushioning bones in joints wear down, leaving your bones rubbing on each other.
Ouch! Osteoarthritis usually shows up in areas of the body you use most often. Think neck, lower back, knees, shoulders, toes, and the base of the thumb.

The second type of arthritis is ***Rheumatoid arthritis*** or RA. This is not the same as OA because it's an inflammatory condition. It rouses your immune system into action, but not in a good way. Instead, it confuses the immune system, inspiring it to attack the tissue lining your joints. As a result, you will have sore, stiff, and swollen joints if you are suffering from Rheumatoid arthritis. In addition to this, the condition comes with nasty side effects (just as nasty as joint pain), including fatigue, poor appetite, and fever. Remember we mentioned that making some wise changes could reverse and relieve joint pain and arthritis symptoms? Well, it's true. Below are a few ways that you reduce joint pain right now:

Strength training – exercise and forms of weight training build muscles that support your joints. Low impact exercises (swimming, cycling, walking) can also help strengthen supporting muscles and ligaments around joints. According to Harvard Medical School (https://www. health.harvard.edu/staying-healthy/5-weight-training-tips-for-people-with-arthritis), weight training is an essential part of easing pain, stiffness, and swelling.

Maintain a healthy weight – being overweight puts excess pressure on your joints, making you more prone to joint pain.

Watch what you eat – some foods spur swelling, pain, and inflammation in the body, and other foods have anti-inflammatory effects. Eating more whole foods (by avoiding those all-too-convenient ready-made meals) is a great way to "eat right" and save your joints from unnecessary aches and pains.

Develop a healthy sleep cycle – we all know that sleep plays a vital role in rest and repair. If you're in pain and you have a restless night, the pain seems worse the next day. According to the Arthritis Foundation (https:// www.arthritis.org/health-wellness/healthy-living/managing-pain/ fatigue-sleep/sleep-and-pain), getting enough sleep is a critical element in minimizing arthritis pain. And, of course, we believe the Arthritis Foundation knows what they're talking about!

If you smoke, quit – studies have proven that smoking can worsen both OA and RA pain.

Decreased Range of Motion

Before we talk about the *decreased* range of motion, let's talk about what range of motion is. It's not just a catch-phrase in the fitness world. Range of motion is defined as the full movement potential of a joint. Small children pop up and down between a kneeling and standing position quickly and without a care in the world. This is because their youthful little knees are enjoying a beautiful thing: full range of motion.

When *you* try it out, it almost seems as if your knee goes so far and then decides, "na-uh." And there you are, midair, somewhere between the ground and standing position, trying to lean into a kneeling position awkwardly. Welcome to decreased range of motion. If you speak with a medical doctor, you will learn that joint range of motion references two things:

1. The distance your joints can move
2. The direction your joints can move in

Many things can lead to a limited range of motion in old age, such as muscle stiffness, pain, inflammation, swelling, and fractures. You may be noticing a pattern here; inactivity can be at play! It can also result from medical conditions such as arthritis, cerebral palsy, Leg-Calve-Perthes disease, and sepsis of the hips and other joints. Now for the good news! You can help to delay the onset by regularly practicing exercises based on a range of motion. The correct exercises can also help you rectify and improve your range of motion if you are already suffering the side effects of a decreased range of motion.

LET'S TALK INJURY & ILLNESS AT 50+

You might have been fearless in your youth, but now that you've breached 50, you're almost walking on eggshells. You know, waiting for those slip and fall incidents or muscle strains society deems us fit for now. Many of the bravest men and women of their time almost cave into themselves with fear of injury and illness as they get older. And it's sad to see people succumb to the cliché of old age. Seeing as this is the chapter about sharing secrets, we would like to share a third secret with you.

> *"While injuries and illness are more common as you age, they don't have to be a fact of life."*

Your mindset is vitally important in this one. If you hold up your hands in defeat at the first glimpse of aging and concede that life will now be about injuries, aches, pains, and illness, then that's the life you will probably have. There's a fantastic life quote that goes, "If you think you can or if you think you can't, you're right," and it couldn't be more applicable to aging. You won't get very far with a defeatist mindset, but focusing on the positive and making wise lifestyle choices will put you on the opposite end of the spectrum, which is not sick and not so prone to injuries, by the way.

The secret (a fourth secret – lucky you!) to living a life that's less prone to injury and illness is to ensure your body is strong, fit, and healthy. A strong and healthy body is resilient against injuries and strong when illnesses come looking for a good host. Understanding the most common injuries and illnesses that sneak up on 50+ers is a good strategy for mitigating them. If you know what to expect, you can make the appropriate lifestyle changes – that's the concept, at least.

Common illnesses and injuries experienced after 50:

- Illnesses
- Injuries
- High blood pressure
- Back pain
- Diabetes
- Meniscus tear (common knee injury)
- Heart disease
- Hematoma (solid swellings of clotted blood)
- Obesity
- Rotator cuff injury
- Osteoarthritis
- Pelvic fractures (falls)
- Osteoporosis
- Shoulder Bursitis
- Eye-sight problems
- Tennis elbow
- Hearing problems
- Lower back pain
- Bladder problems
- Cancer
- Depression
- Dementia (not now, but later on maybe)

A scientific review in the Journal of Health and Sport Science in 2019 found that exercise reduces inflammation, lowers the risk of illness, and improves your immune response. This study was based on doing at least one hour of exercise per day. According to DrPH David Nieman, a professor at the Appalachian State University, humans have a limited number of immune cells floating around their bodies at any given time.

These immune cells are typically found in the lymphoid tissues and organs (the spleen is a favorite of theirs) that destroy the likes of bacteria, viruses, and disease-causing microorganisms.

While doing strength training exercises, your body's blood and lymph flow increase as your muscles contract. This increases the number of immune cells circulating the body. Of course, you cannot do strength training once and expect a miraculous result. While you immediately benefit from an immune boost directly after exercising, this does eventually simmer down, and then you have to do it all over again. Nieman recommends daily exercise for best results. You may find Nieman's study in the 2011 British Journal of Sports Medicine quite interesting. In his study, Nieman found that people who did moderate exercise at least five times a week for three months reduced their chances of getting a common cold by more than 40%. You can read more on this study here if it tickles your fancy: https://bjsm.bmj.com/content/45/12/987.long

But that's all about how strength training can boost your immune system and help you ward off pesky colds and illnesses. How can strength training help you avoid the relatively long list of injuries you can experience after 50? We found an interesting study published in the National Library of Medicine. In summary, this is what the study's findings were:

- Strength-training overcomes frailty and weakness.
- Doing strength training 2 to 3 days per week improves muscle strength, builds muscle mass, and preserves bone density.
- Strength training reduces the risk of osteoporosis.
- Strength training reduces many chronic disease symptoms, including arthritis, heart disease, type 2 diabetes.
- Strength training improves sleep and reduces depression.

That really says it all, but if you want to do a bit of reading into the study, you can find it here: https://pubmed.ncbi.nlm.nih.gov/14552938/

EXERCISE CATAPULTS QUALITY OF LIFE

"Quality of life" is a term we start to hear quite a lot as we near the big 5-0. It's almost the catch-phrase of the era; the 45-50 era, that is. In fact, this quality of life thing becomes even more pertinent as we near 60 and beyond. We're all getting a lot more interested in how much quality our life will offer us in our older years. Now that we're getting older and we have more time to do the things we want to do while we're also a little less agile, we're worried about how comfortable we're going to be and how much enjoyment we're going to, well, enjoy. And for all intents and purposes, this is a very valid focus for our thoughts. If you've been worried about your quality of life, you're not alone in your thinking; in fact, we've been there. We worried that as empty-nesters, our lives would become a blur of one night phasing into the next, eating convenience microwave meals, and watching game shows on television. We feared that our only hope of fitness activities was to wait to reach 60 to join the local 60+ bowling team. Luckily we rekindled our love of sport and fitness and never fell victim to the "You're getting old, just accept it" mindset. And we're welcoming you to do the same because strength training and exercise stand to improve your quality of life greatly.

We probably don't need to refer to a study to provide evidence of this one. It goes without saying that exercise, especially strength training, will promote better heart health, improve your natural energy levels, increase your flexibility, and make you stronger. You will be bending and crouching as required with minimal effort; you will be more than capable of picking up boxes or items of furniture that are heavier than five pounds, and you'll be able to keep up with your energetic grandkids (mentally and physically). Doesn't that sound like the quality of life you're after? Then to add to it, the cherry on the top, so to speak, you'll be digesting your food better, sleeping better, and looking physically better too. This is true quality of life in every sense of the phrase!

FIND YOUR REASON AND GO FOR IT!

If you're even vaguely like the rest of us older folk, you may have found yourself approaching the idea of getting fit and healthy many times but soon revert to old habits. As the famous quote says, old habits tend to die hard, and that's true when it comes to getting back into fitness. It's hard, you feel sluggish, and it seems to take so long to see results that you become demotivated and hopeless. You may find yourself saying, "I will start fitness and strength training next week," or "I don't have time to work out daily," or "I'm too old to start exercising now." All of these are just excuses provided to you - by you - to give up on yourself. This is why having a *reason* is imperative. When you have a reason for doing something, it becomes easier to stick to it. For people to be motivated, there has to be some sort of goal or reward in the end, and you can set those for yourself when you decide what your reason is.

If you really give it a lot of thought, you will realize that you cannot change for someone else. You can't have the mindset of "I will start strength training because my husband wants me to," or "I will start exercising because I have an hour free on Tuesdays." Instead, you need to have reasons for wanting to exercise and do strength training. You have to work on finding a reason or a "why" to get excited about strength training. You want to reach your goals and push onto even higher and more rewarding goals. You don't just want to be able to pick up and cuddle your two-year-old granddaughter – you also want to be able to keep up with her. Having a powerful set of whys is the most essential step in changing.

We've included a few of our why's/reasons to help inspire you to make your own list.

- To become stronger to avoid injuries
- To keep up with the energetic grandkids
- To look and feel better (confidence and self-esteem)
- To slow down the effects of aging
- To get the most out of this next phase of life
- To keep illnesses at bay

Now that you have a decent overview of the illnesses and injuries that may tackle you in your 50's and the importance of staying strong after 50, it's time to page over to the next chapter that digs a little (okay, a lot) deeper into the benefits of strength exercises.

2

THE BENEFITS OF STRENGTH EXERCISES

Now that you're 50+, the last thing you want to do is waste your time on things that don't work. Social media and your groups of friends are awash with all the latest fads and diets. There's a lot out there claiming to be the real deal. So how are you to know what works and what doesn't, especially on a machine that's older than 50? That's the thing – you don't. The best thing to quell your fears is to look at the statistics and reliable sources. But, unfortunately, and we are sorry to say, a lifestyle magazine claiming that an all-cabbage diet is the secret to eternal youth and flexibility is **not** a reliable source.

> *"Strength training BEFORE 50 will make you fit and strong, but strength training AFTER 50 will downright change your life."*

Let's consider one quick study before we get into the nitty-gritty of the benefits of strength training. According to reports by the US National Library of Medicine and the National Institute of Health (both reliable sources, by the way), men and women need strength training more as they age to stay mobile and able in everyday activities. They also say that the main strength training goals for 50+ers are to minimize muscle mass loss and the resulting loss of motor function. The study results also recommended that older people train three to four times per week for the best results. Strength training will keep you strong, healthy, and moving comfortably. We can't really argue with that, can we? And if you want to, we suggest you do a bit of reading in their report first, which is available here: https://www.ncbi.nlm.nih.gov/pmc/articles/PMC3117172/

What we know:

- Maintaining a range of motion as we age is imperative – this is non-negotiable!
- Neglecting range of motion maintenance will result in the shortening and tightening of your muscles, which doesn't sound comfortable at all.
- We all want to keep our muscles strong, flexible, and healthy for as long as possible.
- When muscles are regularly trained, they are ready to jump into action when needed without any pesky injuries setting in.

BUILDING YOUR STRENGTH

Let's jump into the expected (and guaranteed) benefits of strength training for you. At the risk of sounding far too obvious, strength training builds strength. You might have guessed that strength is vitally important when you're heading past your 50th year. In another report released by the US National Library of Medicine and the National Institute of Health, it states that physical exercise has a beneficial effect on various age-related conditions, including the following:

- Osteoarthritis
- Falls (balance)
- Hip fractures
- Cardiovascular disease
- Cancer
- Diabetes Mellitus
- Osteoporosis
- Respiratory diseases
- Obesity
- Overall decreased functional capacity
- Reduced independence (when unfit, you need more help with things)

- Cognition

If you're eager to read the full report, you can access it here: https://www.ncbi.nlm.nih.gov/pmc/articles/PMC4365421

With all of this info in mind, it becomes obvious (again) that strength training is a good idea! One of the bits of info that stood out to us the most (as empty-nesters) was the mention of "reduced independence." Talk about a sensitive topic for us aging folk! Of course, we don't want to become a burden on our children and loved ones as we get older. Yes, they may say that we could "never be a burden," but we know better, don't we? If we need help for every physical thing (think picking things up that have fallen or carrying a chair from one room to another or, heaven forbid, becoming unbalanced and falling more often), it's going to feel like a burden – to us at least. The whole "reduced independence" thing was a severe motivating factor for us. We wanted to be *those* old people. You know, the ones that younger people talk about in awe, saying things like, "wow, there's no way your parents are nearly 60!" And because we started strength training, we *are* those older people!

GOOD FOR YOUR HEAD (COGNITION)

We tend to focus a lot of our energy on our bodies and don't give enough thought to our minds. Unfortunately, as we get older, pesky mental diseases and conditions claw their way towards us. While it is certainly one of life's more uncomfortable things to talk about, we really need to broach the topic. Dementia, Alzheimer's Disease, and general poor cognition all want a piece of your brain as you get older. While you cannot avoid it entirely, as sometimes genetics is involved, you can lower your chances of such conditions getting a firm grip on you by keeping your mind just as fit and healthy as your body.

Here's the good news! Regular strength training positively affects a 50+ers cognition. In 2016, a study on the effects of strength training on cognitive performance in older people was carried out, and the findings were quite interesting. You can read up on the study here: https://www.ncbi.nlm.nih.gov/pmc/articles/PMC4896469

In this study which ran over three months, 29 older people participated. The objective was to verify the impact a resistance/strength training exercise program could have on an older person's physical condition and cognitive capacity. The participants were divided into two groups:

Group 1: This was the control group where simple monitoring of physical and cognitive abilities was carried out (no exercise included)

Group 2: This was the strength training group where each participant was exposed to an exercise program as follows:

- 12 x upper and lower body exercises (3 sets of 10 each) with one-minute intervals between each exercise.
- They repeated the program three times per week using 2.3 kg dumbbells for upper limbs and their own body weight for lower limbs.

Now, you're probably wondering what this has to do with your mental capacity (cognition). And the answer lies in the study's findings. Each participant had to complete the **Montreal Cognitive Assessment** questionnaire after three months. This questionnaire assesses if cognitive abilities have improved at all or remained the same over a period of time. Here's a peek at the entire study's findings:

- Upper body strength showed a standard of 58% improvement
- Lower body strength showed a standard of 68% improvement
- Cognitive capacity increased by 19%

When you consider that these are the results after just three months, it makes you wonder how improved you will think and feel after a year, doesn't it?! With increased upper and lower body strength and a sharper mind to boot, there's reason to believe that strength training can (and does, trust us!) enhance your quality of life. This brings us to our next point.

ENHANCE YOUR QUALITY OF LIFE

If you do strength training for nothing other than to improve your quality of life, you will still be doing a great thing. Strength training provides so many health benefits that it's hard not to enjoy your life more once you're familiar with it and use it to your advantage. Imagine a life where you can get up from sitting on the floor unaided. Imagine heading to the local grocery store where the stairs to the entrance don't daunt you. Imagine walking on a narrow, uneven sidewalk and being absolutely confident that you're **not** going to wobble over, trip or fall. And after that, imagine leaving the grocery store with all your groceries in arms – no need for a younger person to help you carry it all.

This sounds like a good quality of life, but the truth is that many people over 50 don't have that quality of life. They struggle to get up from the sofa, not just the floor. And they fully rely on banisters being available when there's an uneven path or a flight of stairs to deal with. And even worse, they cringe at the thought of their four-year-old grandson running full tilt into their arms because they're not strong enough **not** to fall over. This doesn't have to be you. In fact, with strength training, this **won't** be you. Before we move swiftly along to the next point, let's consider a quick summary of the ways strength training enhances the quality of life:

- Reduces risk of falling
- Burns fat
- Improves daily energy
- Sharpens the mind
- Busts boredom
- Keeps you on your feet and away from embarrassing stumbles (balanced)
- Keeps osteoporosis at bay

LOOK GOOD AND FEEL GOOD!

As we breach the border of 50, most of us develop a habit of letting ourselves go, don't we? And then, one day, you're walking down the sidewalk and catch a glimpse of your reflection in a shop window, and you're filled with immediate self-loathing and embarrassment.

"How on earth did I get this flabby?" Or "What the heck, is that **me?**" might be the thoughts swishing your mind moments later. The harsh reality is that, yes, that is you. But there's some good news too – you can make vast improvements if you're willing to put in the work. Now, we aren't talking about liposuction and botox. While those are options for some people, we would prefer to steer you towards a more natural path.

First, it's imperative to tell you that it's normal to start feeling uncomfortable with the way you look as you get older. Think about it; you have never seen yourself in this older state before, and for many, it's a difficult phase of life to accept. In the first place, you're already feeling bad or awkward about the way you look, so you **could** be looking at your reflection a little too critically. In the second place, you don't have to settle for old age. You can do a bit of moving (and shaking if you wish) to get your body into its best possible state. You can be 50+, yes, but you don't have to look or feel it. Here's how strength training improves your looks and feelings:

- It melts fat
- Regular practice helps you maintain a healthy and sustainable weight
- It develops muscle tone (which looks great on men and women!)
- It improves posture (thanks to strengthening muscles)
- It boosts energy levels (which puts a confident pep in your step)
- It promotes the production of endorphins (which leave you feeling good about yourself)

PROMOTE HEALTHY ORGAN FUNCTION

We all hear the horror stories, don't we? You know, the ones about people we were in school with suddenly developing colon cancer, battling a degenerative respiratory condition, being tortured by seeming incurable restless leg syndrome or similar? These issues speak to incorrect functioning and poor health of organs and, of course, lifestyle choices. Of course, you cannot go back and right the lifestyle choices of the past. Still, you can reduce your chances of becoming another victim or statistic by making better lifestyle choices now. And you guessed it; strength training is on the top of our list of better lifestyle choices. When it comes to healthy organ function, here's how strength training helps:

Reduces anxiety and relaxes muscles (goodbye restless leg syndrome).

Increases blood circulation, thus delivering more oxygen to organs and helping them do their jobs a bit better.

Lowers the risk of colon and kidney cancer – according to a study published in *Medicine & Science in Sports & Exercise*, people who do strength training each week are 22 to 25% less likely to develop colon cancer. The same study showed a moderate reduction in the chance of developing kidney cancer. You can read more on the study here: https://journals.lww.com/acsm-msse/Fulltext/2019/09000/Weight_Training_and_Risk_of_10_Common_Types_of.7.aspx

Improves heart and lung functionality – when your muscles are strong, there's far less demand on the heart allowing your lungs to process more oxygen with less effort. The heart can do its job in fewer beats!

DETER THE WEARING DOWN OF CARTILAGE

Most people 50+ wrongly assume that cartilage wearing down is a fact of life that comes from too much wear and tear. Because of this assumption, they also believe that exercise will cause further wearing down of cartilage and so avoid it. But what if we told you that is entirely untrue? You may argue that arthritis is a form of wear and tear, and that alone is evidence that consistent use of a joint can lead to wear. We beg to differ. If that were the case, then right-handed people would have more painful arthritis in their right hand, right? Now you're thinking, aren't you! Studies have proven that exercise does not negatively impact the wearing down of cartilage unless you are exercising on an injured joint. Now, we aren't suggesting that you head out for a 5-minute mile run when you have osteoarthritis in your weight-bearing joints (think the knees, lower spine, and hips, for instance), as this will merely aggravate your symptoms. What we are saying is that slow, steady, and purposed exercises – such as those in a well-thought-out strength training program – can be just what your body needs to increase bone density and improve muscle strength without wearing down your cartilage.

IMPROVE RANGE OF MOTION

If you've ever seen an older person struggling to reach a product on a higher shelf at the supermarket because they just can't seem to extend their arm fully, you have witnessed a limited range of motion in action. Limited range of motion is a nasty little side effect of old age, but like many other symptoms and side effects, you can reduce its impact exponentially with regular maintenance. If you see somebody 50+ moving fluidly, as if they have no joint or range of motion issues whatsoever, it's probably because they never stopped moving.

Let's explain that.

As the body gets older, it's going to hang onto the functions it does most often. For instance, your legs are used for walking, and you often walk – so there's no issue there, but you don't often squat or reach out for things! With each year that passes that you don't squat down to pick something up or fully extend your arm to reach for things, the less 'essential' that movement becomes and the less familiar the body is with that movement. It's almost as if you start to stiffen in those areas, but we all know it's a lot more scientific than that.

The point is that if you don't squat, stretch or practice picking up slightly heavy things, it will negatively impact those movements and the full functionality of the joints involved. Strength training is a form of maintenance. It helps all your joints and muscles practice their full range of movement, and when that range becomes slightly limited, you can use strength training to reverse the adverse effects.

BOOST AGILITY AND POWER

Let's start with some definitions.

Agility: being able to speed up, slow down, stabilize and change directions with the correct posture quickly.

Power: the maximum amount of force or resistance the muscles can exert on an object.

Now let's think about what these two things mean in terms of real life. Walking the dog, running after your grandkids, jumping up with excitement when hearing good news – these are all things that require agility. Standing firmly on your feet when your grandchild runs into your arms, pushing a lawnmower, or catching something heavy as it falls – these are things that require power. And newsflash, you're not going to get the type of agility and power you need on a treadmill. Now, don't get us wrong, we're not saying that treadmills are out. We're just saying that treadmills and elliptical machines, and pedal bikes, for that matter, place no emphasis on transverse or frontal planes of motion. You may get fit and quick, but whether you will get agile and powerful is questionable. As you get older, your physical workouts should focus on exercises that promote stability in *all* planes of motion. This can be done by carrying out movements at varying speeds and multiple body positions – in short, you can do this with strength training. Strength training develops the muscles and their strength to improve both agility and power overall.

Strength Training Improves Endurance

A lot of people think that endurance is all about speed. They think that endurance in exercise or life is about doing things faster and faster with more precision. And while this is *part* of endurance, it's not what it's all about. Endurance is also about having the energy, strength, and power to do certain things/exercises longer without tiring. Do you know when your grandchild wants to run up and down the garden path again and again? Yup, you need endurance for that. That's just one example – you can surely come up with many more. Think about activities and exercises that you often find yourself getting tired really quickly in. With a bit of an endurance boost, you can do these things for longer without feeling fatigued.

Here's the good news, strength training, when it is done correctly – and by that, we mean the correct exercises, the right amount of sets and reps, with the correct weights and appropriate rest intervals – can dramatically boost your overall endurance. The exercises do this by increasing the amount of force that your muscle fibers produce, and it's only able to do this by strengthening your muscles in the first place. When the muscles exert more force and are more robust, they can repeat this motion over and over without becoming fatigued.

Strength Training Improves Balance and Stability

Because most of us don't remember learning to walk and because after that, balance just seemed to come naturally to us, we forget all the things that we need balance for in life. Well, here's a reminder! You need good balance and stability too (yes, you need to be firmly planted on your feet) for:

- Walking

- Leaning over to look at something or tie your shoelaces
- Getting out of a chair
- Standing on tiptoes to see something
- Carrying plates of food

What creates balance? This is an interesting one to think about, especially as we have already covered the fact that your muscle strength diminishes as you age. Okay, we gave that one away! Your muscles play a large role in balance and stability, along with other things like the snippets of info sent from your eyes to your brain, your joints, and even your ears have a little something-something to do with it. Just knowing this makes it quite evident how the effects of aging can cause balance and stability to deteriorate. Now, let's consider how strength training can help you maintain good balance and stability. Strength training involves strengthening the muscles that help keep you in an upright position. The primary muscles that your body uses in this process are your leg and core muscles. With a well-designed strength training program, you can strengthen your leg and core muscles and, in turn, improve your overall stability while preventing falls.

BOOST YOUR METABOLISM

Metabolism is a sensitive topic for many people, especially those who feel their metabolism isn't fair to them. So first and foremost, what is metabolism? It's just one of those fancy words for the chemical process your body goes through when it converts food to energy. Understanding that definition may give you a good idea of why some people blame weight gain on their metabolism. If your metabolism is sluggish, your body won't convert food into energy quickly enough, which means that your body won't burn the energy but rather store it. Uh oh, that's terrible news for your waistline!

The reality is that as you get a little older than 50 (probably a bit before, too), your metabolism slows around 5% each decade. Yikes! Does that mean that nature's against you, so you're doomed to gain weight and become a blob? No, it doesn't. It simply means that you have to move a bit more and start making healthier, low-calorie nutrient-rich food choices. What is strength training's role in your quest for a speedier metabolism after 50? Well, strength training boosts the metabolism –

that's its role. While practicing strength training exercises, you will actively burn calories.

Building strong muscles doesn't just help you burn calories while you are working out, though. Healthy, well-worked-out muscles even burn calories while they are resting. In fact, studies show that strong muscles burn around 50 calories per day per pound (1/2 kg) of muscle, whereas fat cells only burn around three calories per day per pound (1/2 kg) of fat. This, for us at least, is an excellent reason to start strengthening those muscles!

PROMOTE A POSITIVE MINDSET

Let's talk about your mindset for a bit. Are you one of those 50 year olds with a scowl on your face making grumpy comments about the state of things whenever there's the opportunity? Or are you the type of 50 year old that people enjoy being around because you have happy and positive energy? Who you are as a person, how you feel about life, and how you interact with the world around you all come down to your mindset. What you think will ooze out of every pore of your existence. To avoid becoming that grumpy old man or woman who lives down the road that the neighbors make a wide berth around, you have to do things that promote a healthy and happy mindset. You need to stop dwelling on the negative and start incorporating activities into your life that get you in an excellent mental and emotional space.

Exercise has been proven to promote a positive mindset; in fact, it's one of the most effective strategies for promoting positive thinking. So how does it do this? Exercise releases endorphins, and you know what those are, right? They are hormones that make you feel good. Also, when doing activities like strength training, you have a clear focus on a particular activity which helps to take your mind off other stressful or pressing issues. Getting your mind off the worries you have is almost as good for you as going on an all-expenses-paid holiday of your dreams! Let's take a quick look at how strength training promotes a positive mindset:

- It boosts confidence by making you look better
- Increases energy so you can enjoy your life more
- The endorphins flood you with feel-good hormones

- You have an inner sense of accomplishment as you reach your fitness goals
- It gets your mind off other problems

Now that you have done a bit of reading and better understand the benefits of strength training (and how it can help you) let's move onto Chapter Three: *Send Those Aches and Pains Packing!*

3

SEND THOSE ACHES AND PAINS PACKING

> Welcome to 50. Here's your ailment checklist and a qualifying certificate for the aches, pains, and general discomfort you'll be feeling from now onwards.

Most people envision waking up to this megaphone announcement the moment they peep through their eyelids on their 50th birthday. Reality check! That is all in your head. Well, let's rephrase that. It's all in your head and linked to how much effort you're willing to put into staying fit and spry well into your golden years.

Of course, when we say "how much effort," we're not expecting you to kill yourself with physical exercise. Effort is relative. By that, we mean that when you do five squats after living a squat-free life for twenty years, those five squats are a huge amount of effort. But after practicing squats for three months, you will be flying through four sets of ten squats hassle-free (little to no effort – get it?). And when we say it's "all in your head," we're referring to your mindset. Approaching 50 with a positive mindset is vital. You also approach getting fit with a can-do attitude and a mindset that doesn't buy into the idea that the years you have left will be dedicated to mitigating aches, pains, and other uncomfortable old-age realities.

Now, let us clarify.

A large part of turning 50 and developing aches, pains, slowness, and all the other ailments you're sure will afflict you in your developing age is determined by what you think *in your head.* No, we are not detracting from your very real ailments, aches, and pains. But what we are saying is that your mindset plays a large role in just how severe these symptoms and ailments are to you. While we won't say too much about the power of the mind (which is **really** powerful, by the way), we will present you with a story that made the New York Times. Presenting you with the story of Mr Wright, who we think is a miracle in his own right (no pun intended!). This is a story that we love sharing with others because it illustrates the power of the mind.

The story of Mr Wright is really all about the placebo effect.

*(According to Healthline, the placebo effect is when an individual experiences a physical or health improvement after receiving a bogus treatment. They also say that one in three people are lucky enough to experience the placebo effect. That one person could be you. In fact, we're willing to go out on a limb and say it **will** be you).*

Mr Wright (it's not his real name, by the way, the head honchos of the studies decided to protect his identity by giving him a fake name) was diagnosed with advanced stages of cancer in 1957. There was very little hope for him as they found tumors, some the size of oranges, plaguing his body.

When Mr Wright was hospitalized, he was given his golden ticket to the afterlife – he only had a few days left to live. Naturally, Mr Wright was distraught and, of course, resigned himself to the fact, as he was bedridden and riddled with aches, pains, and all the other things that come with advanced cancer.

While in hospital, Mr Wright just happened to hear a big media announcement about scientists stumbling upon (as they do) a drug called Krebiozen. While this mere horse serum had been around for some time, they had now discovered that it could fight the good fight against cancer, and they suspected it would win! They announced that trials on the drug would begin shortly.

The media excitement got Mr Wright just as excited too. He wanted that treatment. He **had** to have it. He felt as if it was his last hope. So he begged and pleaded to have it. Unfortunately, Mr

Wright wasn't considered a viable candidate, already being on his deathbed and all. However, his pleas and insistence could not be ignored, and eventually, it was decided that he **could** receive the treatment.

Things already weren't looking particularly good for Mr Wright when the treatment program began. He was unable to walk and very weak, but he was hanging on for that new treatment. The day eventually rolled around – the drug had arrived at the hospital and when the doctor administered the very first injection. Mr Wright's gratitude was abundant.

On the other hand, his doctor suspected he might return to a grim finding on Monday – he did not think that Mr Wright would survive the weekend. On his return, a surprise was waiting for him. Mr Wright was out of bed, walking around, laughing and joking. More astounding was the fact that his orange-sized tumors had miraculously disappeared.

The drug was obviously **good.** Better than good. It was the cure to cancer!

And off Mr Wright went to continue living his life.

You probably already know that it doesn't end there. Mr Wright was cancer-free and living life to the fullest when he just happened to read a published report that none of the patients in the trial had experienced a change in their cancer (well, except for Mr Wright, that is). The report also said that the medication had been deemed a failure. He was shocked, appalled even.

What came next? Mr Wright had a mammoth relapse. He was bedridden and riddled with cancer once more. This rather extreme turnaround was of particular interest to his doctor, Philip West. He could tell that Mr Wright had lost all hope. Mr Wright believed that the treatment he received would only lead to his ultimate demise, and there was no telling him otherwise.

Do you see where we are going with this? **Power of the mind.**

Mr Wright initially believed that he would be cured, so much that he was the only patient to recover entirely from cancer after his first treatment. Unfortunately, he also believed fully in the subsequent report. The report only came out months later, but it was enough to convince himself that he was still sick. And because he believed he was sick – he was.

Dr Philip West couldn't stand to see this placebo effect negatively impacting Mr Wright, so he told a little white lie (one we won't hold against him). He told Mr Wright that the drug he had received was merely the wrong version and that a new super-strength version had been released. He was soon to administer the new drug, and he would once again be cured.

Dr West did administer that injection, except unbeknown to Mr Wright, it was only water inside the syringe.

And guess what happened? Mr Wright was once again miraculously cured.

Unfortunately, it wasn't a happy ending for Mr Wright. The placebo effect worked a real number on him. Two months after his 100% recovery (for the second time), the study trials released a definitive report which in short said "Krebiozen **does not** work," and just two days later, Mr Wright, who was free from tumors and illness, died.

We probably don't have to explain the message behind this story. What you think is what you experience. If you expect to have backache and think about it consistently, you will have a backache. If you think you can't do it, you won't be able to do it. If you think you will be consistently ill and full of aches and pains, well, there's every reason why you *will be*, because you *believe* it. A paper released by the Scientific American Mind thoroughly covers the Mr Wright study, how subconscious cues work, the expectation of relief, and the mind's power. If you're interested in doing more delving into the power of the mind and Mr Wrights story, you can find the information here: http://web.as.uky.edu/statistics/users/rayens/A&S100_Resources/PlaceboStudy.pdf

Since Mr Wright's story has been doing the rounds in the medical and scientific fields, a great deal of research has been done into how thoughts, beliefs, and desires impact us physically. New brain imagery techniques have shown that the brain uses a plethora of biological mechanisms to transform a mere thought, belief, or desire into an agent that actually changes the tissues, cells, and organs within the body. This tells us everything we really need to know about just how powerful having the right mindset can be.

The point, ladies and gents, is that at 50+, you cannot afford to have a negative mindset or buy into the misguided belief that the years to follow will be plagued with aches and pains. If you have the right mindset and keep physically fit, you can escape those aches and pains and lead a healthy, active, and comfortable lifestyle. This all really speaks to having good mental health, which plays a major role in aging comfortably. But where do you even start with that? Developing good mental health isn't something you can't just decide to do. You can't wake up tomorrow and say, "I am going to have good mental health now," and suddenly experience it. It takes some practice, just like strength training. Most people know by now that the number one way of developing good mental health is through exercise! Practicing strength training will do wonders for your mindset. Imagine seeing yourself transition from a creaky, achy, stiff 50+er to a strong, capable, and fitter version of yourself. That's good mental health developing as you work out – trust us, we experienced it, and we know you will experience it too.

Other ways you can develop good mental health include:

- Practicing self-care (taking time to do the things that you see as a treat)
- Surrounding yourself with positive people
- Daily journaling about the *good* things in your life
- Learning something new (courses, classes, or asking a family member to teach you something)
- Finding hobbies

Physical Aches & Pains Looking for a 50+ Host

We all know that aches and pains are out there, and they find people who are 50+ the perfect hosts. Aches, pains, and discomforts are the top reasons why so many 50+ers avoid exercise, but ironically they are the very reasons why you should be doing exercise in the first place. If you already have aches and pains, now is the time to make a change. You can activate change by understanding the pains (and aches) and adjusting your mindset and lifestyle to mitigate those issues before they ever become a problem. Until you break the cycle, nothing in your life will change. And don't worry, even if you feel it' too late, it's not. Even if aches and pains have already got you in their tight and uncomfortable grip – you need to know that they are no match for strength training. Let's consider the various aches and pains that usually come looking for people 50+.

EVERYDAY BACK PAIN AND SCIATICA

"I'm just getting old" is probably one of the most over-used sentences in the vocab of 50+ers experiencing a minor ache or pain. One of the most common everyday aches and pains is backache. A 58-year-old man may struggle out of his chair and immediately clutch at his lower back as he shuffles out of the room, saying, "Ah, I'm getting old," almost like some kind of excuse for having back pain. He may believe that he can't go for long walks because he has a sore back. He cannot head out for a jog or do any form of weight lifting because it will just make his back worse. This is the biggest misconception people have. If you have backache, you shouldn't avoid exercise; you should embrace it! He may go on to live the next twenty years with a progressively sore back, saying that same sentence over and over without ever realizing that being over 50 does not mean you have to settle for backache. Because no one ever tells him and because society is so busy shoving the whole "you're old now – retreat to your sofa with a book and knee-blanket" message down our throats, he may never know that by doing simple back stretching and strengthening exercises, he can actually eliminate that pain from his life. That old man could be you – let's hope it's not!

Here's the thing about backache; most of it is mechanical. That sounds a little strange, so let's explain that. It simply means that most backache experience is merely from day-to-day use that can lead to overload. It's not that your back is weak, but if it were stronger, it would be able to handle everyday stresses and not get achy along the way. If you have sciatica, your pain is caused by irritation, inflammation, and nerve compression in the lower back.

The best way to keep everyday back pain and sciatica at bay is through exercise. And that's not just us saying it. In fact, the information comes straight from Ted Dreisinger, Ph.D., who is also the associate editor of **The Spine Journal.** You can gather more of Ted's advice at the following link: https://highintensitybusiness.com/dr-ted-dreisinger

As it turns out, exercise relaxes the muscles, increases blood flow, and reduces inflammation and irritation, which can spur healing. Also, strengthening the muscles leads to a stronger back that can handle everyday lifting, carrying, bending, and standing with greater ease. The National Health Institute tells us that taking to your bed dramatically when backache shows up and lying around until it settles down is counterproductive. It can worsen the problem. At the first sign of backache, you should start walking. A 15-minute walk twice a day would go a long way to easing those muscles and relieving the pain. If you're prone to lower back spasms, stretching can help. You should incorporate a few stretches into your morning routine. Which stretches work best? Here are some firm favorites.

The back-pocket stretch This is a good one to try out. You can do this by standing and placing both hands behind you, almost as you are going to slide your hands into your back pockets. Look upwards and arch your back. This will nicely stretch out your lower back muscles. Do at least 8 to 10 of these each morning.

Press-ups

These aren't everyone's favorite, especially if you struggle to get up from the floor, but they are *effective.* To do this, lie on your stomach, placing your hands on the floor shoulder-width apart as if you are about to do a press-up. Leave your legs lying flat on the ground with your toes extended (do not stand on your toes).

Now, simply push your upper body upwards while allowing your lower back to sag downwards. Push your hips into the ground (it's probably best to use an exercise mat for some padding). Hold this position for a few seconds and then relax before repeating it. You can also repeat this stretch 8 to 10 times each morning.

If you see your doctor about back pain that you experience while standing and he says the term "extension syndrome," don't fret. It's not as scary as it sounds. Extension syndrome is backache caused by all the things you probably spend most of your life doing. By that, we mean sitting in a chair for hours without the right back support. It can also be caused by standing with your knees in a locked-out position.

Naturally, you might think that a sore back while standing is a bad sign and that if you start to get active, it's only going to get worse. This is simply not true. Strengthening and stretching your back muscles will make them stronger and more flexible, leading to improved comfort and less pain. By the way, you don't need a doctor to determine if you have extension syndrome. You can test your body out and see for yourself, but it requires lying down. Lie down on your back on a flat surface with your legs fully extended. Remain this way for half a minute and then raise your legs by bending your knees, so your feet are now flat on the ground. Wait another half a minute and see how you feel. If your back feels achy with your legs out straight and much more relaxed and comfortable when your knees are bent, you may be experiencing extension syndrome. What strength training exercises ease the pain of extension syndrome? You can actually do the stretching exercises already mentioned above (back pocket stretches and press-ups).

Possible Non-Age-Related Causes of Backache

Often, age is blamed for backache making an appearance when usually it's another cause entirely, only worsened by age. Below is a brief look at some of the reasons:

- **Slouching and slumping** – if you've spent a lot of time slouching over or practicing poor posture, this can be the cause of your backache, regardless of your age.
- **Being overweight** – being overweight can cause your pelvis to tilt in an attempt to stabilize the excess weight on the skeletal system. This causes the lower back muscles to tighten and overwork, which in turn leads to backache.
- **Injury** – past injury to your back can come back to revisit you with a few aches and pains when you get older. You could injure your back in a car accident, a slip and fall accident, or even while playing sports (or working out wrong).

We probably don't need to mention this, but strength training can help you reduce your weight and strengthen your back so that slouching, slumping and injury aches are a thing of the past. The main result you're looking for can be achieved: less or no backache.

JOINT PAINS, CARTILAGE, MUSCLE FATIGUE & CRAMPING

Reading this subheading alone is enough to leave you feeling exhausted. In fact, these are the very reasons why so many people say, "I can't exercise because…" Nobody wants to risk the chance of worsening their joint pain or spurring on the quicker deterioration of their cartilage. Much the same, nobody wants to do *anything* that will leave their muscles feeling weak with exhaustion and cramping searing across various body parts. You're getting older, and you may feel like the days of "overdoing it" are in your past. But what if we told you that avoiding exercise is overdoing it in a way? You're overdoing sedentary and allowing old age to wreak havoc on your body. You've gone into war, and you've surrendered even before you find out that the enemy (old age) has no real weapons, and you really hold all the power. Let's look at why these conditions impact 50+ers and why they shouldn't put you off strength training.

Joint Pain

Your joints have quite an important function throughout your lifespan. They're the proverbial workaholics of the human body as they bind the bones together and protect them from knocks and impacts along the way. As you get older, you may notice a stiffness or achiness in the joints. Alternatively, you might feel grating between the joints or a throbbing sensation. If you're struggling to tell if you have joint or muscle pain, joint pain is usually felt when at rest, whereas muscle pain is primarily felt while moving.

You might experience joint pain and instantly jump to the conclusion that you have arthritis. Note that not all joint pain is arthritis. We have an entire section on arthritis a little further in this book. Arthritis is characterized by inflammation that results in joint pain. If you get joint pain without this hallmark, then the pain can be caused by another reason – or just stiffness with age. We like to think of it as getting stale. You know, as you get older, you stagnate – at least some people do. But we have found that you can thwart that stagnation quite effectively by moving and keeping active. Yes, you *can* have healthy, functional, and pain-free joints for much longer.

Most people get joint pain in their feet, hands, knees, hips, and spine, and it can be different for everyone. Some people have constant pain, while others find that it comes and goes.

What Causes Joint Pain?

If you're 50+ and experiencing joint pain, you're probably ready to scream, "Why, why, why?!" especially when no medical treatment seems to help or cure it long term. The most logical answer to what causes joint pain is that as the body ages, the lubricating fluid inside your joints diminishes, and the cartilage becomes thinner. Ligaments that aren't consistently used become shorter and less flexible (which is the reason behind that stiff feeling, by the way).

How Can You Avoid Joint Pain or Overcome it?

Here's what you don't often read but the studies and evidence are out there if you take the time to research it: many of the changes to joints that are age-related are a direct result of lack of exercise. Remember we just told you that the fluid in your joints diminishes over time? Guess what the best way of keeping that fluid level healthy and moving is! You're probably already thinking it: exercise! Lack of consistent movement also causes shrinking and stiffening of the cartilage, which results in reduced joint mobility. So, avoiding exercise because you have joint pain is counterproductive. You should keep moving and strength training to ensure that you escape the entire joint pain debacle altogether.

Benefits of Strength Training for Joint Pain

Strength training won't cause or worsen joint pain but actually, relieve it. One of the main benefits of strength training is to reduce joint pain. The National Institute of Health released study findings that support this claim! You can read more on the studies here: https://www.ncbi.nlm.nih.gov/pmc/articles/PMC3606891

Strengthening exercises loosen stiff and achy joints leaving them with more comfort and increased mobility. While strength training loosens joints, it also strengthens muscles allowing them to be more flexible and thus putting less pressure on the joints. When your muscles are strong and flexible, they carry the load and relieve your joints of a lot of strain and tension.

Cartilage

Cartilage is a connective tissue that ensures the joints move fluidly. It does this by coating the bone's surfaces within our joints and cushioning the bones when bumps and impacts come along. If you start to get older and notice that you have a lot of cartilage loss, it may be the cause of underusing your joints. Recent studies have shown that exercise can rebuild cartilage and maintain it too. That said, studies also show us that strengthening the bone that lies beneath the cartilage is a better idea. This ensures that the bones can handle increased pressure and impacts.

A good way to also protect your cartilage is by strengthening the ligaments, muscles, tendons, and nerves that surround the joint and its cartilage. Lack of exercise can lead to cartilage deterioration because your joints and the surrounding cartilage are designed for movement. They are not designed for a sedentary lifestyle. By incorporating the right exercises and techniques, you can keep your cartilage healthy. While running is said to have a protective effect on cartilage, low-impact strength training is known to strengthen the entire joint, including the cartilage, muscles, and tendons, especially if you are already suffering from joint pain when you decide to get active again.

Muscle Fatigue

Unfortunately, both men and women lose muscle mass and go through hormonal changes as they get older. That's acceptable – after all, we are entering an entirely new phase of life. It's a phase where we no longer require the hormones of the past. We need a fresh set, thank you very much! Age brings with it degenerative changes to the neuromuscular system, which means strength and power become illusionary memories of the past. Diminishing muscle mass is the process of the muscles becoming smaller and also a bit weaker. Why does this happen? Well, to be honest, it's primarily due to a lack of exercise. If you don't use your muscles, they do not need to be big and strong. So, as your muscles diminish and your hormones dwindle, something else happens. Your muscles start to get tired whenever you do something that used to be deemed completely normal in your youth! You pick up and carry something relatively heavy and find your arms getting a little shaky just three minutes in. You feel like your muscles aren't holding up their end of the bargain. Here are the common tell-tale signs of muscle fatigue:

- Muscle soreness
- Shortness of breath
- Localized muscle pain
- Twitching muscles
- Trembling or shaking (especially in the arms and legs)
- Cramps in the muscles
- A weak or slipping grip

OVERCOMING MUSCLE FATIGUE

Many 50+ers avoid exercise because they get tired quickly. Their muscles are weak, and fatigue sets in after a few reps. They start to believe that they *can't* exercise or feel like it's too much effort. Here's a little secret for you – just because you feel tired now, it doesn't mean that you're always going to feel that way. If it's not caused by a serious health condition other than aging, muscle fatigue is something that can you can mitigate. Great news, right? We thought so too.

When we first decided to 'get back in the fitness game,' our muscles were not what they used to be. We could no longer just hit the road running or lift and move weights or sports equipment on a whim like we used to. Just swinging a golf club or hitting a tennis ball can become tiring for aging muscles that are rarely worked out. Our first day back on the court was followed by an evening of stiffness, aches, pains, and ouches. We worried that *this was it.* Was this how life 50+ would be? Should we give up on trying to get back into our sports and fitness? We're glad we didn't give up because we noticed that our muscles slowly but surely picked up the pace as we persisted. We got stronger and more flexible, and what once caused our muscles to give up and have a bit of a shake suddenly became what one can only aptly describe as "easy-peasy." After doing a span of research and using ourselves as test subjects, we found what works to overcome muscle fatigue in your 50s.

Here's what we *know* works:

- Hydrating and eating a healthy diet
- Stretching before and after strenuous activity
- Doing slow, low-impact muscle strengthening exercises
- Increase your endurance (steadily increasing exercise intensity over time)
- Resting between exercise sets and ensuring sufficient recovery time between exercise days

Strength training is the best way to start building muscle strength and mass steadily over time without overdoing it. Slow and steady progress is just fine, and you will be so glad that you did it when you're no longer puffing and panting after a few minutes of strenuous activity.

Cramping

Of course, no one wants to work out if they cramp when they do. But what if we told you that by doing the *right type* of exercises regularly, you would no longer cramp? Would that make you more interested in trying out some exercise? The thing with cramping is that it often sets in without warning, and it's downright uncomfortable. And to make it worse, many people over 50 experience sudden leg cramps even if they aren't exercising. No wonder people want to avoid exercise! They don't want to risk the cramps making an unwanted appearance. The common symptoms of legs, arms, and other muscle cramping include:

- Contractions in the muscle
- Sudden involuntary tightness of hardness of the muscle
- Relief can only be achieved by waiting it out or forcefully massaging the cramping muscle
- Pain lasts for a few seconds up to a minute
- Often, cramping is blamed on old age. Old age seems to be the scapegoat for many conditions. The reality is that cramping can happen for several reasons.

Some of these are listed below:

- Overworking the muscle too soon
- Sitting for long periods without moving
- Underworking the muscle
- Stress/anxiety

Various health conditions:

- Kidney failure
- Dehydration
- Anemia
- Cirrhosis
- Diabetes
- Diarrhea
- Nerve Damage
- Osteoarthritis
- Thyroid issues

Regardless of the symptoms or causes, muscle cramps can be dealt with in the same way. Below are a few ways in which cramping muscles can be relieved not just immediately but over the long term. First and foremost, exercise is an excellent way of minimizing the impact of cramping on your body. When you exercise, the brain releases endorphins which block pain receptors and leave you feeling good. Even if a cramp does come along, you're bound to experience a less severe version of it. Stretching is an excellent way of keeping muscle cramps at bay too. Focus on stretching morning and night and before and after exercises. You will notice that your muscles become more flexible the more you stretch, which goes a long way toward building healthy and robust muscles that are free from cramping.

Body Fat

"I'm too fat to exercise" is probably one of the worst excuses we have ever heard for someone avoiding exercise in old age. Body fat is not just an unattractive thing (no body-shaming here, by the way), but it's also a dangerous thing. According to Harvard Medical School (read more here: https://www.health.harvard.edu/staying-healthy/abdominal-obesity-and-your-health), excess body fat has serious health consequences. Here's why:

- Excess fat is associated with high levels of LDL (bad) cholesterol
- Diminishes the body's responsiveness to insulin and even lead to diabetes
- Carrying excess body fat is linked to heart attacks and strokes
- Excess body fat can cause high blood pressure
- Fatty liver disease results from excess body fat
- Excess body fat spurs on cancer
- Depression often results from excess body fat

Having excess body fat puts additional strain on your bones and organs. If you're overweight, you're putting stress and strain on the body. But why do we put on excess body fat as we age? Unfortunately, as the body ages, fat tissue decreases, making it easier to pack extra fat on. You may find that you're forty-something the one year, eating and exercising well, having a normal weight with a healthy body fat level, and then a few years on you're 50-something and doing the same amount of eating and exercising, but suddenly you're packing on the weight. Becoming more sedentary as you age is not going to help this predicament. It's just going to worsen it. Of course, you don't want to suffer from the above-mentioned health conditions, so what do you do? The top recommended ways to obliterate excess body fat as you age include:

- Making healthier food choices
- Getting enough sleep (yup, sleep is essential to fat-burning)
- Exercising (get that heart rate up)
- Strength training (a muscle-building mass burns fat)

You have already learned that strength training improves muscle size, strength, and function. It also boosts metabolism, which helps with burning body fat and calories. The great thing about strength training is that as your muscles strengthen, they will continue to burn more calories and fat even after your workout.

Arthritis

We already spoke about arthritis and joint pain. Arthritis is always joint pain, but joint pain is not always arthritis. This is because arthritis is joint pain characterized by inflammation. We'd like to tell you something about arthritis that most people don't know. Arthritis is not a health condition that discriminates against 50+ers only. It's a disability that affects people of all ages. In fact, in the United States, more than 300,000 children have arthritis. Yes, it's more common in older people, but it's not an affliction reserved for older people only. This brings us back to having the right mindset. If you're gearing up for arthritis in your old age, just think about this: you may not have to deal with it at all. You are not **destined** to have it. That aside, older people do get it, and that's not something to overlook. What is arthritis? We've already established that it's inflammation of the joints. It can plague one or multiple joints, and pinpointing what type of arthritis it is can be tricky as there are more than 100 different types. While this is true, most people experience one of two common types: Osteoarthritis (OA) and Rheumatoid Arthritis (RA).

Some of the most common symptoms of arthritis include:

- Joint pain
- Swelling
- Stiffness

- Decreased range of motion
- Redness of the skin by the affected joint

Rheumatoid Arthritis can be a bit more brutal by including all of those symptoms along with tiredness and loss of appetite. It can sometimes even progress to anemia. Now, if you have arthritis, you may immediately think that you need to rest your weary joints and avoid movement and exercise at all costs. Well, that's where you're doing things wrong. If you see a doctor about your arthritis, he/she may give you some medications to try and recommend that you take pressure off your joints by using a cane, walker, or similar. Doctors using advanced treatment methods may also advise that you use physical therapy to improve joint mobility and reduce pain. Physical therapy for arthritis involves exercises that strengthen the muscles around the affected joint. There we go again – strength training saves the day!

CHRONIC CONDITIONS

We've heard it time and again; "I can't exercise because I suffer a chronic condition." That's just not true. Exercise boosts endorphins, strengthens the immune system, and gets the body fighting fit. Surely *this* scenario plays out more positively than someone who sits around allowing their chronic condition to ravage them? Exercising when you have a chronic condition is fighting back! But wait, what exactly are the chronic conditions that affect 50+ers most commonly? Here's a brief list as supplied by the National Institute of Health (you can read their report here: https://www.ncbi.nlm.nih.gov/pmc/articles/PMC4880619/#:~: text=Chronic%20diseases%20include%20cancers%2C% 20cardiovascular,and%20intestinal%20problems%20(2))

- Cancers
- Respiratory diseases
- Diabetes
- Hypertension
- Cardiovascular diseases
- Strokes
- Mental disorders
- Arthritis
- Rheumatism

- Dental problems
- Deteriorating eye-sight
- Gastrointestinal problems

If you read articles online or in newspapers, you may have come across several sources that claim exercise can lower your risk of developing a chronic condition in the first place. Even if you have a chronic condition already, exercise plays a major role in effectively managing the condition and its symptoms. And we're not saying that strength training is the only answer.

Let's take cardiovascular conditions as an example. Cardio workouts can actually help prevent heart disease. But if you find that you have high blood pressure and high cholesterol (which are markers of heart problems), doing cardio exercise can help you reduce those problems and reduce your chances of having a heart attack or stroke. Now, let's consider strength training. Strength training builds stronger muscles and healthier joints, improving mobility as individuals age.

But that's not all that strength training does. When it comes to thwarting chronic conditions, strength training can minimize arthritis pain and improve control of type 2 diabetes. And if you're prone to slip and fall incidents, the improved flexibility, strength, and range of motion that strength training provides can put an end to those pesky slips and falls. Here's what else strength training can do to help people with chronic conditions:

- Improves sleep
- Protects and improves brain function
- Develops and maintains bone density
- Boosts the immune system
- Boosts injury recovery

So, if you think that your chronic condition is a reason to avoid strength training (and other forms of exercise), think again. It's the very reason you **should** start strength training – as soon as yesterday!

Poor posture isn't just something that makes younger people look sloppy. It's something that can create a wealth of discomfort for whoever has been indulging in it. Some of the common disadvantages of poor posture that impact 50+ers include:

Incorrect Spine Curvature

If your spine is in the correct alignment, three primary curves give the spine an "S" shape. Over time and as you get older, consistent poor posture can result in those natural curves changing. When these curves aren't as they were designed, you will find that all the pressure from your body's weight is in all the wrong places on the spine. If you think about it, the spine's designed to absorb shocks and impacts, but it's difficult for the spine to carry out this function if you have a poor posture. This means that an injury can end up being quite serious.

Backache

When your back isn't in the correct posture, it leads to strain on the lower and upper back that it otherwise wouldn't have. If you slouch forwards, this puts pressure on your shoulder blades, and if you find that you have pain around your tailbone and neck pain too, the chances are that you're not sitting up straight. Other disadvantages of poor posture include:

- Headaches
- Neck pain
- Disrupted sleep
- Poor digestion (poor spinal curves can compress organs and slow down digestion)

So, where does strength training come in? Well, you might think that your symptoms of poor posture are good reasons to avoid exercise. After all, it's natural to assume that these symptoms will only worsen if you put any sort of pressure on the back and spine at all. But that's where you're wrong. One of the first recommendations made for correcting poor posture or managing the symptoms is physical therapy. And do you know what they do in posture physical therapy sessions? They do *strength training*. By strengthening weak muscles in the back and spinal area, the pain of poor posture can be greatly reduced while improving your overall posture too. Once the muscles are stronger, the physical therapist will assist the patient with improving the range of motion. Which is something that we already know strength training can achieve. So why wait until you get to the point where you need to work with a physical therapist when you can do preventative and maintenance strength training at home?

Bone Density

Dwindling bone density is a scary prospect for anyone. If you have low bone density, you won't feel any pain as your bones become thinner. However, you will be at greater risk of breaking bones if you happen to fall or bump a limb hard on something. Why does low bone density happen? As you get older, the body gets to work reabsorbing calcium and phosphate from the bones. As you can imagine, this doesn't leave your bones much to work with, so they become weaker. If your bones lose density and mass to a severe point, low bone density can become osteoporosis. 50+ers with low bone density can take a calcium supplement. This won't boost your levels but can provide maintenance so that your body doesn't absorb all of your bone's calcium supplies. If you go this route, take your calcium supplement with vitamin D to promote better absorption.

Another great way of responding to poor bone density is to incorporate strength training into your weekly routine. One thing we know is that stressing the bones actually increases bone density and if you've been doing it all your life, lucky you, you have a very slim chance of getting osteoporosis. You might be wondering how exercise can increase bone density. It's quite a simple concept. The bones in your body are living tissue. They respond to the experiences they have. If you place force on your bones, they will start getting denser to handle the pressure and impact better. Your bones are constantly adapting, which means just like they can become denser when you work them out, they can lose density when you don't. If you're leading a sedentary life as a 50+er, you're at risk of diminishing bone density!

Internal Organs

Many people believe that their internal organs get old and creaky when they breach the 50's border. People get gastrointestinal disturbances, liver disorders, breathing issues, and even heart conditions. The internal organs are who we are. Without them, we would not exist. So if you feel that you have internal organ ailments, you may think that you need to "take it easy" and give your organs some time out. Again, this is the wrong approach. There's overwhelming evidence that exercise promotes internal organ health. We all know that the heart is one of the most critical organs in the body. It pumps blood around to all the essential organs, and that's why you have to keep it fit and healthy. If it gets clogged arteries, high blood pressure, or slows down for some reason, you're in trouble. While cardiovascular exercise is often punted as the only form of exercise for the heart, the truth is that any exercise that increases your heart rate is good for your cardiovascular health. And strength training will definitely increase your heart rate.

Another way that strength training can positively influence organ health is by keeping your body weight healthy. Being overweight and carrying excess body fat puts your organs under undue pressure. Of course, exercise also helps boost the body's ability to eliminate toxins – just another way that strength training can keep your most vital organ, aka the entire body, healthy!

Injuries

Past injuries and the fear of getting new ones often put people 50+ off the idea of exercising. Perhaps you have an old injury that's imposing pain on you now in your more senior years. Or maybe you're worried that you'll start exercising and develop pain and injuries along the way. First and foremost, if you do strength training and learn the correct way to do that (yes, we cover that in this book), there's a very slim chance that you're going to injure yourself. And if you have a past injury, you may be interested in knowing that strength training can reduce the pain you're experiencing.

It's important to point out that strength training develops strong muscles, improves balance and stability, and encourages better form. This means that you will be able to perform exercises without injury, and if you do happen to injure yourself, your fit and healthy body will recover pretty quickly. In addition to this, your stronger muscles, improved form, and newfound stability/balance will ensure that you experience fewer slip and fall incidents and are far sturdier on your feet when walking on uneven surfaces.

If you're genuinely scared of possible injuries, consider this. Some studies (you can read more on them here: https://www.ncbi.nlm.nih.gov/ pubmed/3633121) prove that strength training inspires the strengthening and growth of muscles, ligaments, tendons, cartilage, bones, and connective tissue. With this type of strengthening and using the correct exercises, you won't just improve your body's performance but decrease your risk of injury and exercise-related pain.

Stress

Many people are bogged down with stress. They're so stressed that they can't think straight. And just because you are 50+, it doesn't mean that your stress magically disappears. You may have work stress if you're still working; you may have family stress, social stresses, or be worried about your finances. There's no telling what can and does stress people out. But what we do know is that stress kills. It can have a dramatic impact on your health. Stress left to run amock in your body can present you with physical, emotional, behavioral, and cognitive disadvantages. As a result, you can experience long-term consequences, including the following.

- Mental health issues (depression, personality disorders, anxiety)
- Heart disease, high blood pressure, heart attack, or stroke
- Weight gain
- Gastrointestinal problems, ulcerative colitis, and irritable bowel syndrome

It can also leave you struggling with headaches, insomnia, irritability, and more. Here's the good news! Strength training can help you reduce stress levels and minimize all of these associated symptoms. The biggest challenge will be convincing yourself that you *do* have time for exercise and actually giving it a chance. After just a few weeks, you will notice a major turnaround in how stressed you feel. As a form of exercise, strength training reduces stress hormones in your body (these are cortisol and adrenaline). In addition to this, strength training boosts the production of feel-good endorphins, which are known as mood elevators and natural pain killers. It's hard to feel stressed when you're on such a natural high!

BODY ALIGNMENT

You may think that body alignment and posture are the same things, and while they play into each other, they aren't entirely the same thing. Posture is all about the spine and how you sit and stand. It's all about having the correct "S" curve that we spoke about earlier. Body alignment is about how the head, shoulders, spine, hips, knees, and ankles align with each other to impact how you sit, stand, and move around. When all of these features are in alignment, it means there's no undue stress on the spine or any other part of your body. You know the saying "you're in alignment" – well, that's kind of what it means – everything is perfectly in its place.

Many of us have little to no idea about how to move our bodies so that they are in the correct alignment. For instance, you may sit on a chair and bend down to the ground to tie your shoelaces when the correct way would be to raise your leg while keeping your back flat. Now, imagine an entire lifetime of making small motions just like this one, wrong over and over. Now you've got a good idea how *out of alignment* most of us are. And that, of course, can lead to aches and pains when we are older.

That doesn't mean that all hope is lost, of course. Strength training cannot change the past, but it can help you improve your current alignment and reduce any pain you may be experiencing from past alignment issues. It does this by building up the muscles, bones, and other supporting tissues in the lower back and the rest of the body. When these are stronger and more stable, it improves your posture and leads to better body alignment throughout the day. The result? You have no reason to fear the pain and discomfort that comes from poor body alignment!

Now that you've got a much better understanding of the common conditions that scare 50+ers of old age *and* getting active, it's time to move on to learn more about how strength training impacts your core and takes your body strength, fitness, and health to the next level.

Let's page over to Chapter Four: *Why Core Strength is a Priority.*

4

WHY CORE STRENGTH IS A PRIORITY

Why is core strength so important? Actually, why is it so important when you're passing 50 and probably have no intention of posing for swimsuit calendars or strutting your stuff, mid-section fully exposed, on the beach (or anywhere, really!)?

The truth is that having a strong core is about more than just a stunning set of abs. Unfortunately, most of us only learn this as we get older. Things change a little when you're 50+. Suddenly you're not as stable on your feet as you used to be and movements are a little more deterred than usual. Sadly, these changes sneak up on us. That said, now is the time to tell you the truth about the core. Are you ready for it? The core comprises multiple muscles in the torso. Yes, more than just that elusive six-pack that most workout enthusiasts spend their youth trying to achieve. The core includes a variety of much deeper muscles below the surface. The name "core" really gives it away, doesn't it? It's implying that it's deep inside – in the "middle."

These muscles all work together to do a lot more than craft easy-on-the-eye aesthetics. Their entire design is geared towards supporting and stabilizing your spine, which essentially makes everyday movements easier (or, should we say, more natural). In addition to this, a sturdy and robust core also makes you more stable on your feet. It improves balance, and as a result, you can be less fearful of those pesky fall accidents.

WHAT IS THE CORE & HOW DOES IT WORK?

Okay, so now we have a better idea of the underlying function of the core. It's weird to think of these muscles that we don't intentionally activate managing such an important bodily function! It's one thing to say that it's a set of muscles deep in the core, but what does that even mean?

Let's dig a little deeper.

The core muscles in your body do their work in your pelvis and around the spine. As a result, these muscles can have an impact on your legs and upper body too. You probably think someone who is ultra-strong and powerful must have a strong core. Likewise, you might look at a bodybuilder with inflated muscles and be convinced that he has a potent core, but that's not always the case. Core strength doesn't have much to do with how much power a person has. It's more about how strong that set of muscles are in maintaining a particular pose firmly without getting weak and giving in. In essence, it's more about the durability of the muscle and how much control it has over its movements. When a muscle is strong and in control, it reduces the load imposed on the joints and makes movement easy. If you've ever watched someone with a strong core doing sit-ups gracefully or managing to make a one-legged full-body plank look elegant, it's because they have a strong core. They make it look easy because their strong core muscles make it a lot easier for them to do.

But that doesn't sound like you, does it? Not many people in the 50+ club are found pumping iron or showing off their elegant planks at the gym. And that's okay, but it doesn't mean that you don't need to get a strong core. Having a strong core will do a lot for enhancing your quality of life. How? Well, here's what you can expect to do with *greater ease* when your core is strong and in control of its movements.

- You will be able to sit down on the floor and stand back up again without all the crawling around, hobbling, or grabbing onto furniture items for help.
- A knock from your galloping grandchild will be just that, a knock. It won't send you toppling over because your muscles will be strong enough to counter the impact of the knock and keep you standing firm.
- You will stand up from a chair with greater ease.

- You will sit comfortably at a desk without associated pain.
- Hauling a vacuum cleaner back and forth will no longer be a source of great pain and discomfort.
- You will suffer fewer injuries (if any) and strains when exercising or doing something a little more active than usual.
- And here's one we probably don't want to talk about; incontinence. Some older folk experience problems with this as they get older. It should be comforting (and significant motivation to get started) that having a strong core can strengthen the pelvic floor and surrounding muscles, known to reverse and even prevent incontinence.
- You will be able to easily swing a golf club or tennis racket several times without feeling exhausted.

A strong core stabilizes your body and allows you to move in any direction, even when on the bumpiest path. You can even stand in one spot without feeling like you're going to topple over. And more importantly, you *won't* topple over*!*

WHAT'S SO BAD ABOUT A WEAK CORE?

Having a strong core can provide all the above-mentioned benefits, so what does that tell you about a weak core? One thing that we cannot get away from as we get older is that our bodies age. We can slow down aging and better manage the process, but we can't *stop* it. As part of the aging process – and we're sorry to be the bearers of bad news – your body will go through various degenerative changes. Unfortunately, the spine is often the first to experience negative side effects. Do you know the pain that sneaks up on you, the sudden strange posture, the hunched-over look (scoliosis)? All of these things are thanks to the spine and its function degenerating. And it's not just the bones and joints of the spine, by the way; it's the muscles too.

At the same time, structures of bones and cartilage also go through some changes and become sensitive to wear and tear. This happens because the core is not strong enough to maintain the body in the correct posture. And if you let all of this happen without intercepting the symptoms, it's a pretty fast downhill journey to poor mobility, crooked spinal development, and aches and pains to boot. Remember that song most of us sang as kids? You might even remember the words. (it seems this song is timeless). It went a little something like this:

> "The thigh bone's connected to the ...hip bone. The hip bone's connected to the ...backbone. The backbone's connected to the ...neck bone. Doin' the skeleton dance!"

And that's the underlying message. Absolutely everything within your body is connected, and your core is at the heart of it all. If your core isn't strong and in good shape, many things can start to go wrong. In fact, a weak core can inspire aches and pains all over the boy. For instance, weak pelvic muscles lead to pelvic instability, which can result in knee pain! It sounds weird, but it's true. And when you've got knee pain, it's safe to say that your knee joints are not absorbing the impact of your walking, jogging, running, and similar, and that can lead to neck and back pain too. It all boils down to the core. If the core were strong in the first place, most of these issues would never crop up! You're probably wondering if there's any good news, and there is! A little bit of good news is that you can better manage, overcome and even completely obliterate these uncomfortable symptoms of a weak core by starting to do the correct core strengthening exercises. And before you ask, yes, even scoliosis (curving and rotation of the spine) can be controlled and corrected with the proper core strengthening exercises.

ALIGNMENT AND FLEXIBILITY

When the body is not in alignment, it leads to overworking the muscles. To understand what's happening in the body, let's think of a choir. When a choir practices and each member knows precisely at what pitch and tone to sing, it can sound beautiful – harmonious even. But if the choir doesn't know what it's doing, it can end up sounding like the proverbial cat's choir. Each member will be singing at the wrong speed, in the wrong tone, sounding like an absolute mess. Perhaps with some practice and by being shown/and directed, that cat's choir can become harmonious too.

It's much the same with the muscles in the body. When the body is aligned, it is flexible, strong, and holds all the muscles and joints in perfect positions. As a result, there is no stress and strain on the joints or muscles. The muscles, joints, and all the other bits and pieces in your body are in harmony. When the body is not aligned, the muscles tire out, and the bones and joints start to fuse and mold awkwardly.

Cue the cat's choir. You experience muscular aches and pains because the body pulls in all different directions, which is tiring and exhausting for the average set of muscles. Quite frankly, the body is a mess. But, with some regular and consistent practice and by showing the muscles what they need to do, you can overcome this problem. You can achieve harmony in your body by developing the one area responsible for pulling everything into alignment and ensuring greater flexibility. And yes, that one area is the core!

THE LINK BETWEEN POSTURE AND CORE STRENGTH

At this stage, you're probably wondering why it's your core that's responsible for keeping the body aligned and not your posture. We spend many years being told that posture is the key to good body alignment. But, unfortunately, you're not told the whole story. Posture *is* important for body alignment. It's downright essential, but what you don't know is that core strength plays an integral role in how good your posture is - and how bad it is too. Weak core muscles are the culprit of slouching, protruding your shoulders, or simply sitting and standing incorrectly. When the core muscles are strong, they pull the body into a position (the correct one) that eases the strain on your back muscles. As a result, you can stand up straight and enjoy a healthy posture!

STRENGTHENING YOUR CORE, IN THE REAL WORLD!

What does having a strong core mean for you in terms of real-world value? How will having a strong core improve your quality of life after you surpass the 50 milestone? Below is a look at *some* of the benefits we have seen others experience (and we have experienced too).

The Everyday Stuff

Your core is involved in absolutely *every* movement you make. That said, a strong core can make everyday activities a lot easier, such as bending to tie your shoes or pick up a package, turning in your seat, standing still, getting dressed, or maintaining balance when a dog jumps up on you.

Grocery Shopping & Cleaning House

Do you know how much strain carrying heavy grocery bags puts on your back? What if you didn't have to endure that pain? A strong core will ensure that your back is well aligned and sturdy. With a strong core, you can say goodbye to aches and pains from grocery bag carrying, vacuuming, sweeping, raking, or simply tidying up the home.

Healthy, Strong Back

It's not uncommon for 50+ers to say they have a "bad back," in fact, it's pretty much expected. This is because most people (and we mean around four out of five Americans) experience pain in the lower back at some point in their life. And when someone seeks treatment for lower back pain, they are always provided with a list of exercises that develop strong core muscles. That's because the core is responsible for keeping the back strong.

Sports & Activities

Just because we're getting older, it doesn't mean we have to miss out on the sports activities we've always enjoyed (or enjoyed when we were younger). When you have a strong core, the actions that may currently seem tiring on your body will get a lot easier. Think about riding a bike, hiking, walking, rowing, jogging or even going for a run without experiencing backache, arm strain, or even tired leg muscles.

Avoid Chasing the Abs Dream

Even at 50+, we have seen people chasing after the dream of having rippling abs, and while that's commendable, we must serve a warning. Overworking your abdominal muscles just for aesthetics can lead to injuring the back and hip muscles. Steady and focused strength training exercises that are done correctly and with rests in between are the only type of core exercises you *need* to be doing.

Finally, we've reached the exercise portion of this book. Page over to Chapter Five: *Strength Training at Home* to learn how to warm up and which strength training exercises are best to start with.

5

STRENGTH TRAINING AT HOME

You're all clued up, now what? What can you do with all of the information you have learned about strength training and its positive impact? Now is when we inspire action into you. Get up and do it! Leap into action!

Okay, maybe we should steadily work our way into action instead of leaping into it. If you do anything too quickly, you're only going to injure yourself and delay reaching your fit-and-fab-after-50 goal. We've heard many of our followers say that the exercises they find online just aren't designed for 50+ers. And we agree. Many of them aren't going to inspire much enthusiasm in your workouts because they're difficult to follow and are designed for a much younger fitness group. Much the same, heading to the gym and joining a class with all the "youngsters" is just going to leave you feeling deflated and left behind.

The most important part of this process is realizing that you're kickstarting your body from sedentary into action, which has to be done slowly and steadily. You're young at heart, but your body isn't what it used to be. That doesn't mean it can't be greatly improved, but you have to do so with care. You can't suddenly join an advanced fitness group and expect to keep up. You have to listen to your body along the way too. If you're in serious pain during a workout, slow down, take a break, and make sure you're doing the exercise correctly. To ensure that you're doing the right exercises and movements for a mature physique, we have compiled a selection of strength training exercises that you can do at home and at your own speed. Before we ease into any stretching and flexing (easy now!), let's talk about responsible training.

Disclaimer: You should always consult with your physician or healthcare provider before changing your regular exercise program or trying new forms of exercise. You should not use the book's contents as a substitute for professional medical advice, treatment, or diagnosis. If you have received medical advice that is opposed to the information found in this book (everyone's situation is unique), please do not discard that advice. While we have done everything to ensure that this book provides responsible and safe advice and exercise routines, it is important to practice any of it solely at your own risk. If you have any existing physical disabilities or conditions or have a past injury, seeking the advice of your healthcare provider is first and foremost advised.

Now that we have that out of the way, let's jump into the fun part. This is the moment you start to change your quality of life!

WARM-UP ROUTINE

Before you start doing anything physical, it's important to warm up. Warming up your muscles gets them to relax and become more supple. It also increases the overall flow of blood and oxygen to the muscles, ensuring that they are well-nourished throughout the exercise process. This is important if you want your muscles to perform (and you do). At the same time, a warm-up gets your joints ready to move and enjoy a better range of motion. As a result, there's less risk of injury, and you suffer fewer after-exercise aches and pains (don't worry – all exercise pains lessen the more you exercise). Warm-ups should only be around five to ten minutes long. Below are four warm-up exercises to do:

Back Arch Stretch

- Stand with your feet shoulder-width apart.
- Gently lean back with your hands on your hips.
- Hold the position for a few seconds.
- Gently return to your starting position.
- Repeat 3-5 times.

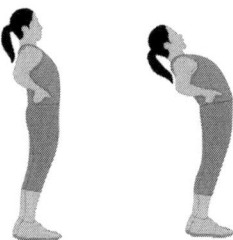

FIGURE 1-1: BACK ARCH STRETCH

Tricep Circles

Loosening and warming up your triceps is an important part of the process.

- Extend your arms directly out at your sides with palms down.
- Keeping your arms straight, rotate them so that you make backward circles with your hands. Do this for 20 seconds.
- Repeat the process, but in a forward direction for 20 seconds.
- Turn your palms to face forward – now pulse your arms backward and forwards as if you are pushing something with your hands. Do this for another 20 seconds.

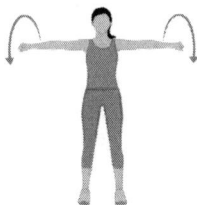

FIGURE 1-2: TRICEP CIRCLES

Walk/Run on the Spot

Of course, you need to get your heart rate slightly up so that it's ready for your workout. You can do this by running or walking fast on the spot. Find a space where you won't bump into anything.

- Either walk or jog on the spot for 20 seconds
- Rest for 10 seconds and repeat the process.
- In total, repeat this exercise three times.

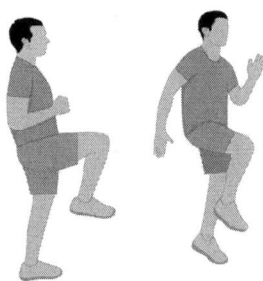

FIGURE 1-3: WALK/JOG ON THE SPOT

Wall Push-ups

Instead of doing a regular push-up, we will do wall push-ups until you have built enough strength to try doing push-ups the traditional way (on the ground). Wall push-ups warm up your arms, shoulders, and chest. How to do a wall push-up:

- Make sure you are just an arm's length away from the wall.
- Position your feet shoulder-width apart.
- Extend each of your arms directly out in front of you and place your hands flat on the wall.
- Breathe in deeply and bend your elbows while you lower your body closer to the wall. While you're doing this, tighten your core and buttocks muscles (this actually helps you to maintain a straight position that's firm).
- Hold the position close to the wall for two seconds, and then push

your body backward with your arms without removing your hands from the wall.

- Do not raise your heels when doing this exercise – your feet should remain firmly planted flat on the floor.
- Do two sets of 10 reps of this exercise.

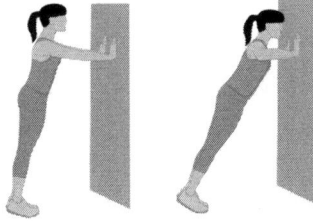

FIGURE 1-4: WALL PUSHUPS

You're warmed up and ready to get started!

Easy Peasy Strength Training Exercises – No Equipment Required!

We've spoken to many 50+ers who feel overwhelmed by all the exercise and gym equipment out there. Yes, the fitness world has come a long way, and there are many things you can buy and use that are meant to make your workout easier and more effective. But here's what you need to know: equipment is *not* essential. You can get a full-body workout that really *works* without using a single item of equipment. The following ten exercises illustrated here make this point quite nicely. Each of these exercises is highly beneficial to both men and women in the 50+ club, and if you do each of them, you will essentially have done a full-body workout. We encourage you to try each of these exercises, even if you think they seem hard. You will be surprised at just how easy many of them are.

Make sure that you have these items handy before you get started.

Exercise mat (the thicker, the better) if you can't get a mat in a hurry, a very thick folded towel can be a good substitute.

Towel (to dry up any sweat, yes, you're going to sweat)

Water bottle (staying hydrated between exercises is essential) take small sips of water when you can throughout your workout. Don't gulp a lot, as it will just make you feel uncomfortable.

If you're exercising outside, make sure that you have sunscreen or a hat to protect you from the sun.

Good pair of exercise shoes, gym floor shoes or running shoes will suffice. Don't attempt to do exercise in your regular shoes as they don't provide sufficient grip or support.

Suitable exercise clothes. Choose clothes that are fitted without being too tight. If your clothing is too loose and baggy, it will just get in the way and make you feel hot. A tee-shirt or vest and sweatpants or shorts (or yoga tights) are suitable.

#1 – Chair Squats

You've already warmed up with a similar version of these, so your muscles are good to go. This exercise builds and improves bone density while strengthening the pelvis. Choose a chair in the house – something that's similar to a dining room chair will work well.

- Position your body in front of your chair, keeping your feet shoulder-width apart with your toes turned slightly outward.
- Extend your arms, keeping them in a parallel position to the floor (keep your arms in this position for balance throughout the exercise).
- Bend your knees while being careful to keep your back straight. Then push your hips back just until your buttocks touch the base of the chair. Do not actually *sit* on the chair even if your body is making requests!
- As soon as your buttocks touch the chair, push into your heels and stand back up. That's one rep.
- Complete 3 sets of 12 reps.

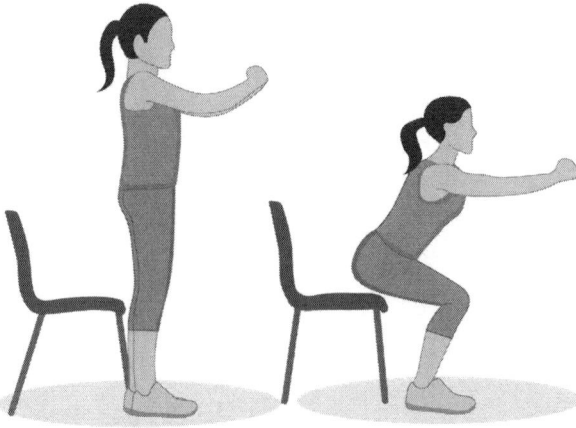

FIGURE 2-1: CHAIR SQUATS

#2 – Standing Calf Raises

Many people forget the calves, but they play a vital role in walking and running. They also play a role in balance. Strengthening your calves is important to provide both endurance and explosiveness. It also improves ankle stability and balance. This is a great exercise for stretching the plantar muscles of your feet.

- Stand with your feet positioned slightly apart.
- Push yourself in an upward position - onto the balls of your feet.
- If needed, stand in front of a table or wall, so that you can support/stabilize yourself by touching the wall/table.
- Hold this position for 3-5 seconds, and then relax your calves so that your feet are flat on the ground again.
- Keep a tall, long spine position while doing this exercise.
- Repeat 2 sets of 15 reps.

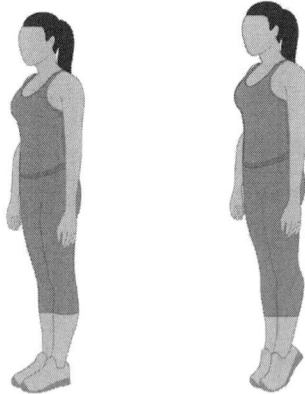

FIGURE 2-2: STANDING CALF RAISES

(Calf Raises continued)

#3 – **Single Leg Version** Once you get more strength and balance in your calves, you can start doing one-legged calf raises. Here's how to do that:

- Stand with one hand gently on the wall or table in front of you for stability.
- Bend your knee and bring one foot up behind you and hold it with the other hand.
- Use the wall or table to provide some more stability.
- Keep your back straight (do not push your buttocks out) and lift your heel off the floor and onto the ball of your foot.
- Hold this position for five seconds and then relax and return to a flat standing position.
- Complete 2 sets of 10 reps for each side

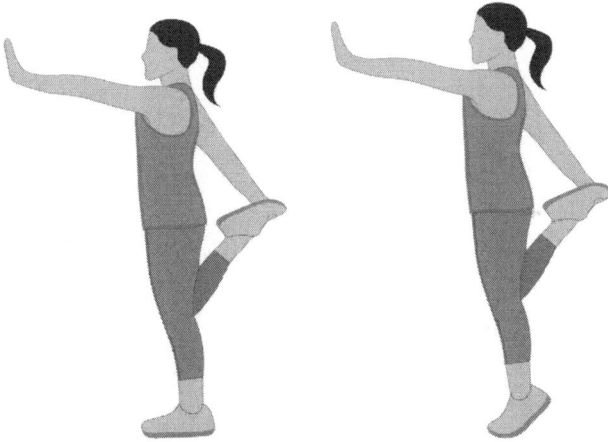

FIGURE 2-3: SINGLE LEG CALF RAISES

#4 –Basic Ab Crunches

This exercise strengthens your core, and is essential for good posture. When doing a basic ab crunch, your abdominal muscles are pulled inward toward the spine. This makes your abdominal muscles tighter and stronger.

- Lie flat on your back using a mat or towel as padding.
- Keep your feet firmly planted flat on the floor with your knees bent. This will create a 45-degree angle behind your knees.
- Keep your upper body relaxed and place your hands behind your head.
- Breathe in deeply and then when you breathe out, slowly tuck your chin in toward your chest and pull your shoulders halfway off the floor (do not sit the whole way up).
- Pause in this position for a second, and then gently lower yourself back down into the start position.
- Repeat 2 sets of 20 times (but if you can, aim for 30).
- It is important that you focus on using your core muscles to lift and raise your shoulders. (don't use your arms and hands to lift your neck).

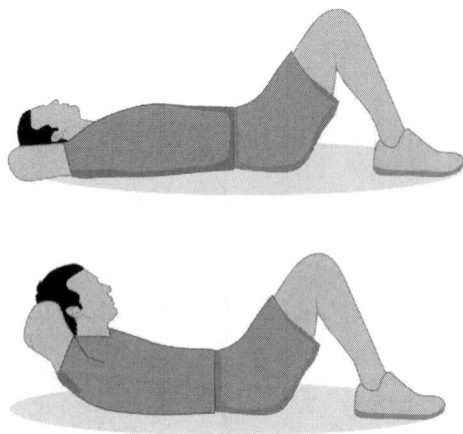

FIGURE 2-4: BASIC AB CRUNCHES

#5 –Hamstring Bridge (single leg)

This is a brilliant exercise for gaining strength in your core, glutes, hamstrings, and lower back.

- On your exercise mat or thick towel, lie flat on your beck.
- Place your feet flat on the ground hip-width apart.
- Lie with your arms straight down by your sides with your palms flat on the ground. Your hands provide stability.
- Extend one leg straight out, and then raise it to point your toes at the ceiling.
- Raise your hips off the mat while squeezing your glutes (buttocks muscles). This will push you into a bridge position.
- Hold the bridge position for 2 seconds, and then lower yourself back down to the ground.
- Repeat 2 sets of 8 reps - for each side.

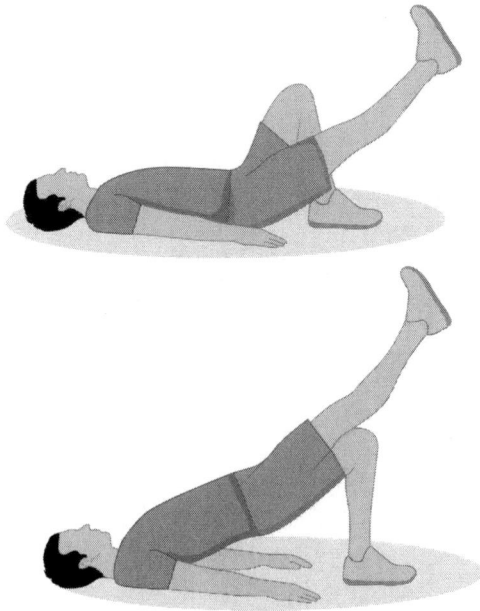

FIGURE 2-5: HAMSTRING BRIDGE

#6 – Modified Push-Ups

A modified push-up is a great option for those who are getting back into fitness. This exercise targets the shoulders, upper body, triceps, biceps, back, chest, and core. Squeeze your ab muscles while doing this routine.

- Start by kneeling on your mat or thick folded towel with your hands flat on the ground, shoulder-width apart. Now, each arm should be fully extended.
- Position your knees back behind your hips so that you are now in a semi-plank position.
- Look directly down. This keeps your neck in the correct position.
- Squeeze your glutes (buttocks muscles) and inner thighs together while keeping the lower part of your body active.
- Gently lower your body down to the floor while ensuring your elbows stay back at a 45-degree angle. Your knees remain on the ground for this exercise, providing stability.
- Immediately push yourself back up into the starting position with arms fully extended. Do 3 sets of 8 reps.

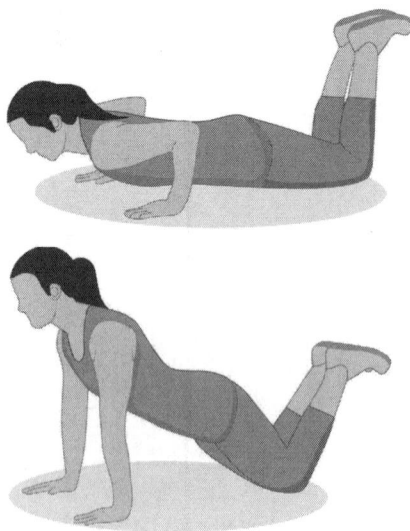

FIGURE 2-6: MODIFIED PUSH-UPS

#7 – (Push-Ups continued)

Once you have mastered the modified push-up, it's time to try a traditional push-up from your toes. Here's how to do that.

- Begin in a high plank semi-position, just as you did in the exercise above.
- Make sure that your hands are shoulder-width apart.
- Slowly transition your legs from a kneeling position to a long extended position behind you, standing on your toes.
- Now your body is in a high plank position with your back and legs in a straight line.
- Lower yourself towards the floor, with your elbows pointing back only slightly. Stop before you touch the ground.
- Breathe out and squeeze your abs while you push yourself back up into a plank position.
- Repeat 3 sets of 8 reps.

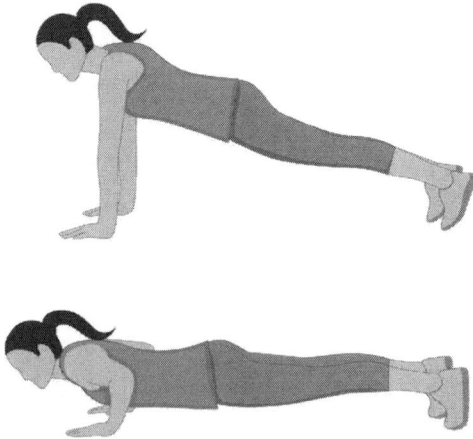

FIGURE 2-7: PUSH-UPS

#8 – Basic Lunges

We like to call lunges our secret to staying stable and agile. These exercises do far more than most people realize! Lunges strengthen the back, hips, and legs. They also improve stability and mobility – two things that become increasingly important as we age. Do this exercise next to a wall or a table (if you need stability).

- Make sure that you are standing with a tall and straight back with both of your feet positioned hip-width apart.
- Squeeze your core muscles while placing hands on your hips.
- Take a big step forward with your right leg.
- Lower your body until your right thigh is in a parallel position to the ground and your right shin is vertical.
- Don't allow your knee position to move past your toes (this would be poor form).
- Now, simply press into your right heel while pushing your body up as you step backward again, returning to the start position.
- Repeat 2 sets of 10 reps -for each side.

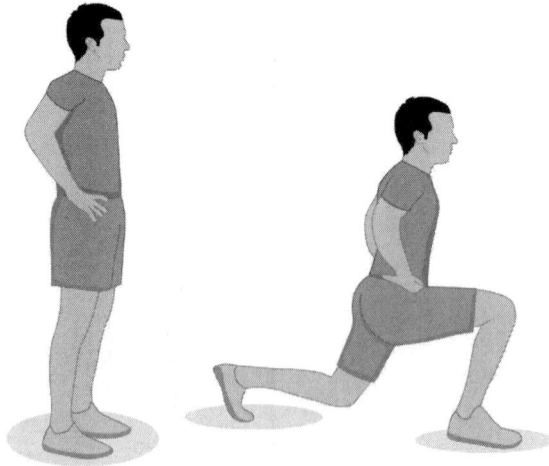

FIGURE 2-8: BASIC LUNGES

#9 - Plank

The plank is a whopper of an exercise because it works out the entire body and comes with many benefits. When you get the hang of planking, it improves both balance and posture while strengthening your core. It develops and strengthens your spine, shoulder bones, joints, and pelvis. But wait, there's more! It also increases flexibility, trims the fat that likes to hang around the belly, and reduces backache. Starting from a kneeling position on your exercise mat will be the easiest for you. It will make getting into the plank position a lot easier.

- In the kneeling position, place your hands with palms flat on the ground directly below your shoulders. Make sure that you take care to spread your fingers wide, as this will help with balance and stability.
- Lower yourself and bend your elbows so that you are now resting on your forearms.
- Slowly extend your legs behind you and balance on your toes.
- Tuck your hip bones forward as if you are pulling your belly button and hips towards each other.
- Hold this position firmly for 30 seconds, and then relax.
- Repeat this three times with 20 second rests in between each.

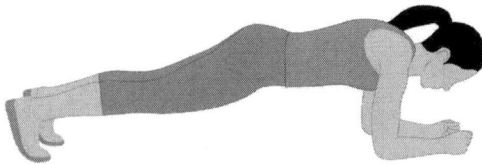

FIGURE 2-9: PLANK

#10 - Ground Tricep Dips

The triceps are a powerful little muscle that most people forget to exercise. Working out your triceps will make all the ground-based exercises easier as it builds upper body strength and stabilizes the shoulder joint. Having strong triceps will also make it easier to play a number of sports.

- Sit on the floor with your hands flat on the ground with palms flat and fingers pointing towards your feet.
- Ensure that your hands placed below your shoulders.
- Extend your legs with your feet hip-width apart, knees bent.
- Keep your chin up while looking directly ahead of you.
- Then, push yourself up to lift your body from the floor without letting your heels or feet do the work for you. Ensure that your arms are doing the pushing.
- Hold your position with buttocks off the ground for three seconds, and then slowly lower yourself to the ground.
- This is a very small movement, but if you do it correctly, you should feel a burn in the back of your arm.
- Repeat 3 sets 10 reps.

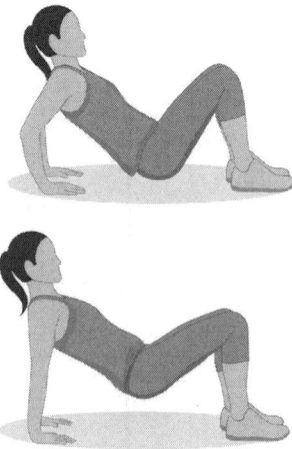

FIGURE 2-10: GROUND TRICEP DIPS

If you're only just getting started with fitness after many years or months of inactivity, complete this set of exercises once. As you progress and get stronger and fitter, you can increase to doing two sets of each. Make it your aim to eventually work up the strength to do four sets of each exercise (four sets of 15 reps for each). Ideally, if you are strength training every second day, you should be able to work your way up to this strength and stamina within four to six weeks.

ADDING FITNESS TOOLS TO YOUR WORKOUT

Using your own bodyweight to do strength training, as depicted in the previous-mentioned exercises, is fine to start with and also just fine for regular exercise. However, there are definite benefits to adding equipment and tools to your workout. We've already discussed dwindling muscle mass and depleting bone density as you head towards 50, and if left unchecked, this will only increase with time.

Adding weights and other items of equipment to your strength training routine will boost metabolism (three cheers for faster weight loss!), gain muscle mass and strength, maintain bone density and boost mental sharpness, too (there's more to think about when there's equipment involved). Weighted exercises also help improve range of motion and overall flexibility. We aren't expecting you to invest in a range of expensive workout gear, but there are tools that we often use because they boost our workout results by making each exercise more effective. Here's a look at our top picks – we recommend you get these!

Swiss Ball (also called an exercise ball, balance ball, or yoga ball) Swiss balls are quite popular strength training tools as they are so versatile. They are used at the gym and at home, and their primary function is to improve balance, strengthen your core, and improve muscle tone and flexibility too. Most 50+ers experience an increased range of motion, a much stronger core, and are sturdier on their feet when using an exercise ball. Stability balls are available in various sizes, and they are both lightweight and durable. They're just filled with air, so you can blow them up manually or use a bicycle tire pump. These balls are great for doing push-ups, bridges, planks, and leg curls, to name a few.

Hand Weights or as they are more commonly called dumbbells, are great for building bone mass, challenging the muscle, and ensuring that you balance strength by equally exercising both sides of your body. 50+ers who include dumbbells in their workouts experience improved balance and coordination, along with increased stability in their joints and muscles. They typically range in size from lightweight to extremely heavy. You only need to think about getting two 3 pound hand weights and two 5 pound hand weights to get started. For men who have a bit more strength, 8-10 pound hand weights should suffice for your strength training. Of course, start lightweight and work your way up as you feel comfortable. Hand weight-friendly exercises include bicep curls, overhead tricep dips, punching, shoulder presses, floor presses, bent-over rows, squats, lunges, and arm raises to name a few!

Adjustable dumbbells and hand weights are pretty much the same things, except with adjustable dumbbells; there's a mechanism included to change the weights quickly and easily by removing weight plates and replacing them with others. This means that you can transition between exercises without having to select different dumbbells each time. If you don't have the space to cater to a selection of dumbbells, then adjustable dumbbells might be better suited to you. One of the advantages of using adjustable dumbbells is that you won't have to keep buying new dumbbells as you get stronger and fitter. Of course, you can do all of the very the same exercises with adjustable dumbbells as you can with hand weights, including bicep curls, overhead tricep dips, punching, shoulder presses, floor presses, bent-over rows, squats, lunges, and arm raises to name a few!

Resistance bands are made from stretchy rubber. They can be looped on other equipment or used on their own. They are great for building strength by exerting force on your muscles. They are used for both upper and lower body strength training.

Most 50+ers who use resistance bands regularly experience improved mobility and flexibility, including more range of motion in their joints. When shopping around, you will find various types of resistance bands ranging in thickness and width. It's important to know that the thicker the band is, the more resistance it exerts, meaning that it's more difficult to work with than thinner bands. The most common bands are the flat ones, and they usually range from Level 1 (the easiest to use) and range up to Level 6 (the hardest to use). If you are just starting out, choose a Level 1 resistance band and aim to work your way up as you get stronger. Some of the exercises you can do with resistance bands include squats, chest presses, bicep curls, lateral raises, leg presses, and seated calf presses to name a few.

BASIC STRENGTH EXERCISES WITH EQUIPMENT

Now we're getting to the exciting part. You're reading to take your workout up a notch by adding in a few items of equipment. This isn't going to make your workout more difficult – it's going to make it more effective.

Here's a sneak peek at a few exercises you can try, and we highly recommend you try each of them out. Just one set of each exercise is okay to start with, but you should aim to work your way up to doing four sets each (that's four sets of 15 reps for each exercise). Later in chapter six we delve into a lot more detail (be prepared!).

Let's get started with some basic equipment!

#1 –Punching/Boxing with Hand Weights

It should come as no surprise that boxing or punching strengthens the core muscles and the back, legs, arms, and shoulders. For 50+ers, this is a great workout because it gets the heart rate up, builds muscle mass, and is a mental challenge too.

- Select a 2-5 pound set of dumbbells.
- Stand with your feet shoulder-width apart while holding the dumbbells with bent arms. The weights should be positioned at shoulder height, and your palms should be facing inward.
- Punch diagonally with your right hand across your body to the left side while keeping your weight at shoulder height. Do this in a very slow and controlled movement.
- Don't hold your torso too firm. Allow your torso to rotate naturally as you punch (be careful not to swing your hips).
- Keep your lower body still throughout the entire punch.
- Repeat this movement on the opposite side. Keep alternating slow punches.
- Repeat 30 alternating punches (15 punches each arm)

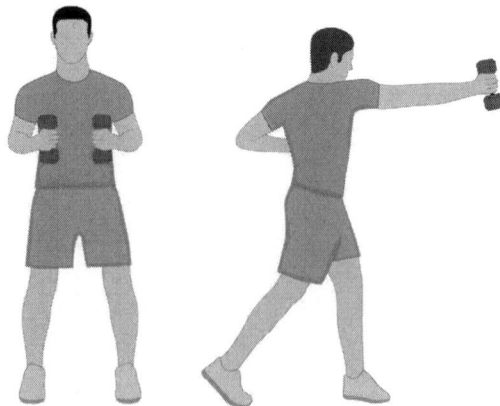

FIGURE 3-1: BOXING WITH HAND WEIGHTS

#2 –Seated Calf Press (Resistance Band)

Calf raises can be intensified while also being made a little easier by using a resistance band.

- Sit flat on the floor with heels on the floor and toes pointed up to the ceiling.
- Sling the resistance band underneath your feet and hold onto each end with your hands.
- Position the band at the ball or middle of your feet.
- Ensure that you keep your back straight and your head up during this exercise.
- Now, pull the resistance band upward as you flex your toes back down towards the ground.
- You can do this fast or slow – whatever works best for you.
- Repeat 2 sets of 12 reps.

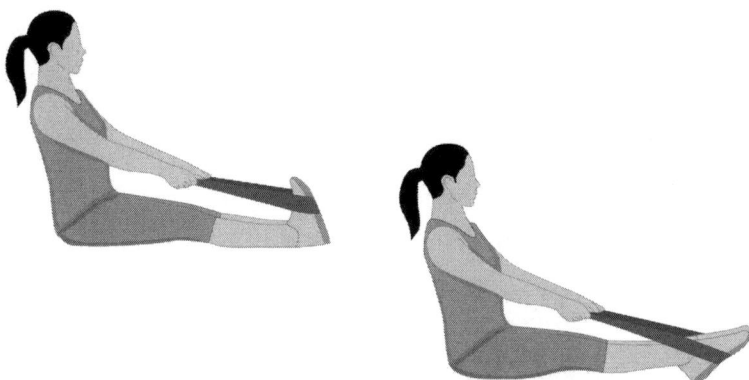

FIGURE 3-2: SEATED CALF PRESS

#3 –Core Balance (Swiss Ball)

Doing core balance exercises will strengthen your core, improve posture, and as a result, improve your overall balance too. A Swiss Ball isn't very tricky to stay on, but it does engage the core to ensure you don't slide off or wobble over to the side. Throughout the exercise, your core muscles are at work.

- Sit on the exercise ball and place your hands to the sides of your head.
- Lengthen your spine (we call this "sitting proud") and push your head up towards the ceiling.
- Keep your feet firmly placed together on the ground directly in front of your exercise ball.
- Now, lift one foot off the ground and hold it in a raised position for 3-5 seconds.
- Lower your foot back to the ground and then lift the opposite leg for 3-5 seconds.
- Repeat this exercise 20 times and alternate each leg (10 raises each side).

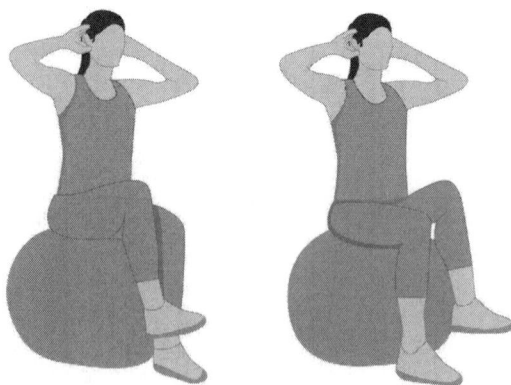

FIGURE 3-3: CORE BALANCE (SWISS BALL)

#4 – Seated Dumbbell Shoulder Press

This is a seated exercise, so make sure that you have a chair or bench handy. Seated shoulder presses take some pressure off the core, but perhaps your core needs a bit of a break at this stage anyway. The seated shoulder press with adjustable weights or dumbbells is great for improving shoulder strength, building stronger bones, and improving your overall stability.

- Sit on the chair or bench in an upright position and hold your dumbbells in each hand at shoulder height. Your palms should be facing away from you.
- Keep your chest pushed up and engage your core for stability.
- Look directly forward throughout this exercise.
- Push the dumbbells upwards until your arms are fully extended towards the ceiling.
- Pause briefly and then slowly and controlled, lower your arms back to the starting position.
- Repeat 3 sets of 8 reps.
- Later, consider moving to 10 reps.

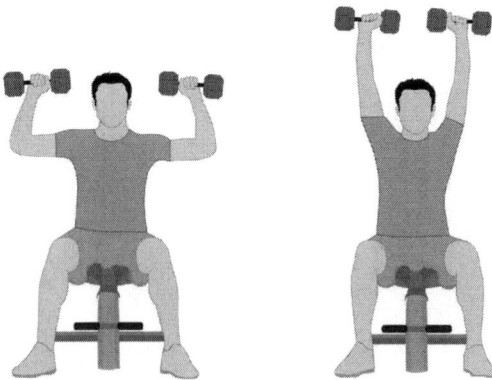

FIGURE 3-4: SEATED DUMBBELL SHOULDER PRESS

#5 –Hamstring Bridge to Curl (Swiss Ball)

You've already done the hamstring bridge without any equipment; now it's time to add a challenging element.

- Lie down on your back on your mat, and raise your legs with your feet directly above the ball.
- With the exercise ball directly below your feet, dig your heels into the top of the ball with your toes pointing forward.
- Place your hands firmly on the ground beside you, palms down, to help with stability.
- Now, lift your hips and buttocks off the floor into a bridge position.
- Then, slowly roll the ball toward your hips by bending your legs at a 90 degree position
- Hold the bridge for three seconds, and then slowly roll the ball back to its original position by straightening your legs.
- That's one complete rep.
- Repeat 2 sets of 10 reps.

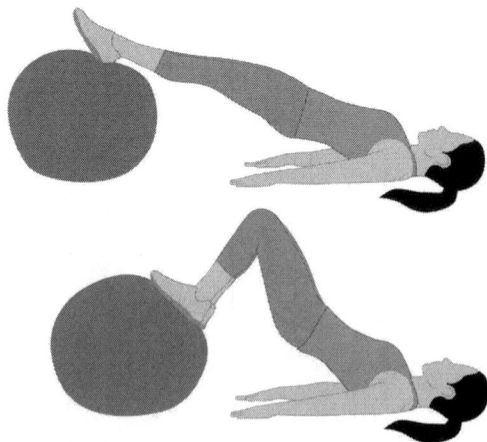

FIGURE 3-5: HAMSTRING BRIDGE TO CURL (SWISS BALL)

#6 –Basic Lunges (with dumbbells)

When you lunge with dumbbells, it helps to tone the arms, strengthen the core and work on your stability too.

- Select a 3 to 5-pound weight to begin with (if you can handle heavier, do it!)
- Holding the weights straight down by your sides or snuggly to your chest with your knuckles almost rubbing, take a big step forward with your right leg.
- Lower your body until your right thigh is in a parallel position to the ground and your right shin is vertical.
- Don't allow your knee to go past your toe (this would be poor form).
- Next, press into your right heel and push your body up as you step backward again, returning to the start position.
- Repeat 3 sets of 10 reps.

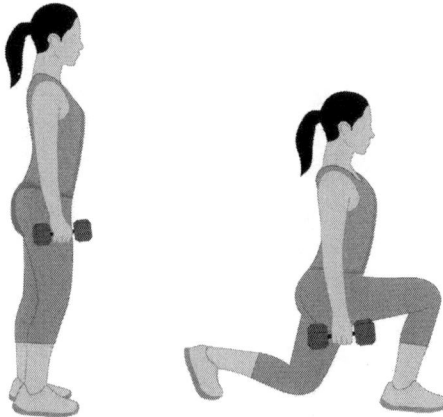

FIGURE 3-6: BASIC LUNGES (WITH DUMBBELLS)

#7 –Elastic Ab Teasers (Resistance Band)

Doing ab exercises with a resistance band effectively builds muscle strength and durability while developing the core.

- Lie down on your mat facing the ceiling with your legs together.
- Wrap the resistance band under the soles of your feet, holding each end at your sides with your hands.
- Now, pull on the band using both hands to pull yourself into a V-sit position (it sounds harder than it is, promise).
- Hold the V-sit position for 3-5 seconds, and then slowly lower yourself (in a very controlled manner) back down to the ground.
- Repeat this exercise 15 times.

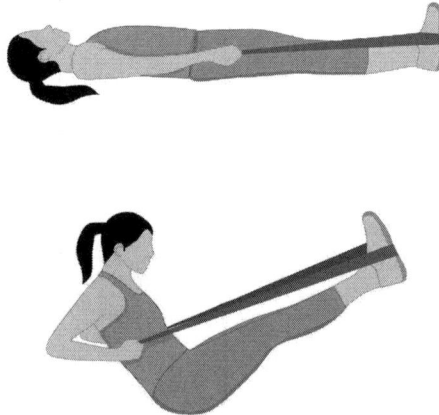

FIGURE 3-7: ELASTIC AB TEASERS (RESISTANCE BAND)

Hopefully, these simple yet effective strength training exercises have excited you as much as they excited us! The above exercises are just a taster of the strength training you will be doing.

Do you know what time it is? It's time to page over to Chapter Six: *Strength Training with Equipment.*

Chapter six will teach you basic exercises that you can do with each item of equipment (hand weights, adjustable dumbbells, resistance bands, and exercise balls).

STRENGTH TRAINING WITH EQUIPMENT

W ell done, you've progressed to the hard bit. This is the chapter where we address exercise from a slightly more complicated approach. Don't worry – it won't always be complicated; it just might *feel* that way initially.

> Jim Rohn, a motivational speaker who is well worth looking up, once said, **"Take care of your body; it's the only place you have to live."** We couldn't agree more.

You spend so much time maintaining and cleaning your home, even to extreme physical efforts, yet when it comes to our bodies, we simply let them dwindle and weaken. Luckily, you're taking steps to put more maintenance time into your real home: your body!

In the previous chapter, we discussed the appropriate exercises and movements to build strength while exercising. We also ran through the various fitness tools that can help to enhance your efforts. In this chapter, you will add to the strength-building foundation you have been working on by incorporating simple tools to enhance and improve your workouts and movements, resulting in increased agility and strength. We have eliminated the confusion of choosing which equipment is best from an ease-of-use and practicality point of view (you're welcome). No one wants a truckload of 'useful' gadgets based on their price tag and popularity alone. We carefully selected the tools we have already mentioned to allow you to do an array of exercises and routines without taking away from your flexibility of choice.

We don't know about you, but just like those easy midweek one-pot recipes, exercise equipment that can be utilized in multiple ways is every bit as tantalizing as that last piece of apple pie! That said, we have chosen four fitness tools that you can use in a wide variety of exercise routines. Without any further ado, let's up the ante, slowly, of course. This next part in the program will see you stronger and healthier, with added body confidence that's sure to put the swagger back in your 50+ step.

SWISS BALL, BALANCE BALL

Incorporating a Swiss ball or balance ball into your exercise routine will help build abdominal and lower back muscles. One of our favorite workouts includes Stability ball crunches, which sound a whole lot tougher than they are. These exercises target muscles such as the transversus abdominis, a vital core muscle; which stabilizes the lumbar spine and pelvis before moving our legs or arms. This is definitely a muscle you want to strengthen if you find you're becoming a little less stable on your feet.

Ensure the balance ball is inflated correctly; check the manufacturer's guidelines, making sure you have not overinflated or under-inflated it (this is an important part to check).

Let's look at how to do the stability ball crunch along with a handful of other exercises that can be done with your balance ball.

#1 – Stability Ball Crunch

As the name suggests, this exercise is based on doing a basic crunch. This crunch movement is what strengthens the abdominal muscles and improves posture, balance, and stability.

- Lie face-up with the ball positioned under your lower back and just below your shoulder blades.
- Your feet should be flat on the floor hip-width apart; this will aid your balance, so make sure it's not just your toes that are touching the floor.
- Simply put, tighten your buttocks and brace your abdomen.
- Put your hands behind your head and slowly raise your shoulders off the ball. Then, tuck your chin inwards to your chest. This is the crunching motion that gets the job done!
- Lower yourself back down onto the ball and return to the start position. That's one rep.
- Repeat 3 sets of 10 reps.

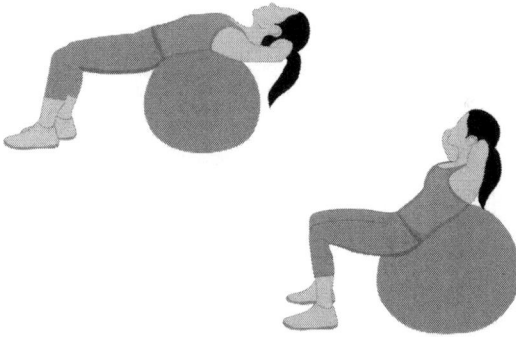

FIGURE 4-1: STABILITY BALL CRUNCH

#2 – Stability Ball Knee Raise

This exercise is brilliant for targeting the core as it works the arms, legs, lower back, and abdominal muscles simultaneously. It also works out the smaller stabilizing muscles that keep you balanced.

- Lie on your back with the balance ball positioned under your lower back and just below your shoulder blades.
- Ensure that you place your feet flat on the floor hip-width apart; this will ensure that you can balance throughout the exercise.
- Squeeze your buttocks and tighten your ab muscles.
- Place your hands behind your head and lift your right foot; bring your right knee slowly towards your chest. Hold for thirty seconds.
- Slowly replace your right foot on the floor, repeat lifting the opposite foot, and hold for thirty seconds. You have now completed one rep.
- Repeat 3 sets of 10 reps.

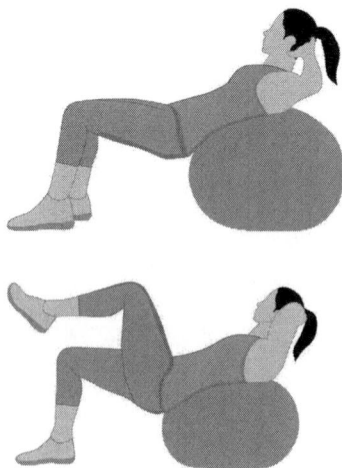

FIGURE 4-2: STABILITY BALL KNEE RAISE

#3 – Stability Ball Bicycle Crunch

This exercise is brilliant for any 50+ers with lower back pain. Not only does it reduce lower back pain, but it also strengthens the obliques and hip flexors, strengthens the abs, and improves overall balance and posture.

- Lie face-up and position the balance ball under your lower back. Make sure it sits just below your shoulder blades.
- Get your balance firmly before moving on to the next step.
- Place your feet flat on the ground, hip-width apart. Tighten your buttocks and abs at the same time while placing your hands behind your head.
- While keeping your ab muscles engaged, raise your right knee towards your chest; at the same time, bring your left elbow towards your raised knee. Don't worry if they don't touch. Do this movement very slowly.
- Lower your right foot and upper body simultaneously and repeat on the opposite side. That is one rep. Repeat 3 sets of 10 reps.
- *Tip: Remember to use your abdominal muscles to lift your upper body. Don't pull up using your back or neck muscles.

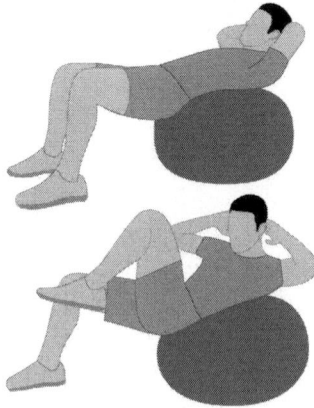

FIGURE 4-3: STABILITY BALL BICYCLE CRUNCH

#4 – Stability Ball Oblique Crunches

Your obliques cross near the side of your midsection diagonally. They run from the bottom of your rib cage to your pubic area. Your obliques help you bend side to side and also assist with waist twisting movements. A strong set of obliques stabilizes and protects your spine. By now, you know how to get into a basic ball crunch position with your hands behind your head. Assume this position and make sure that you're stable and balanced.

- Remember to brace your core and tighten your buttocks.
- Now, crunch up and to the right, lift your shoulder blades off the ball, and rotate your upper body to the right. Note this is the same as a basic crunch but just with a slight sideways twist.
- Slowly lower back onto the ball and repeat the same movement, crunching to the left this time.
- One rep is two crunches, one per side.
- Repeat 2 sets of 8 reps.

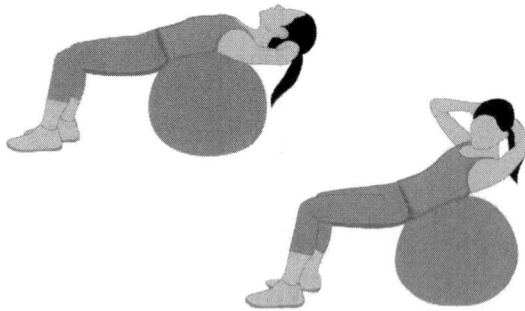

FIGURE 4-4: STABILITY BALL OBLIQUE CRUNCHES

#5 – Stability Ball Hip Thrust

This exercise strengthens your buttocks and legs, which play into overall stability and balance. They're a great exercise for 50+ers who want to maintain stability even on rough terrain.

- Lie on the floor with each of your legs straight and with heels resting on the balance ball.
- Your hips should now be resting on the floor and your arms on either side of you.
- Keeping your core and buttocks tight, raise your hips up until your body is in a straight line.
- Hold this position to 2 seconds.
- Then, let your hips lower back down to the starting position.
- That is one rep.
- Do 2 sets of 15 reps and increase as your strength improves.

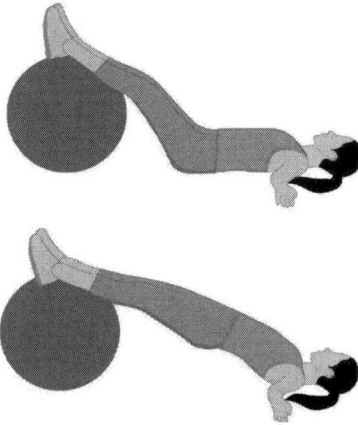

FIGURE 4-5: STABILITY BALL HIP THRUST

#6 – Stability Ball Hands to Feet Pass

This exercise requires some concentration, but we find it a lot of fun. While you are having a giggle at yourself doing this, rest assured that it's strengthening your core and back muscles!

- Lie on your back while holding the ball with outstretched arms as the illustration shows.
- Breathe deeply and tighten your ab muscles.
- Keep your head and shoulders flat on the floor.
- Raise your legs towards your arms, pass the ball from your hands to your feet. You can get a firm grip on the ball with your ankles.
- Exhale as you lower your legs and the ball to the floor and pause.
- Inhale and lift your legs towards your arms and pass the ball back to your hands. That's one rep.
- Aim to complete 10 reps (and increase the number of reps as you get stronger).

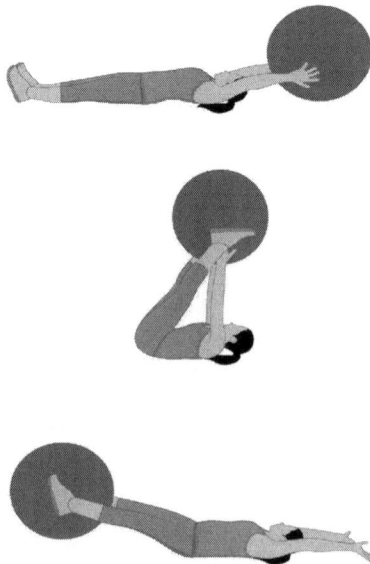

FIGURE 4-6: STABILITY BALL HANDS-TO-FEET PASS

HAND WEIGHTS & ADJUSTABLE DUMBBELLS

* We have included hand weights and adjustable dumbbells into the same section as you can use either option when doing these exercises.

Hand weights and adjustable dumbbells, more commonly called free weights, allow you freedom of movement and aid in a range of strengthening exercises such as the weighted glute bridge, which sounds like something out of a Star Wars movie! But, unlike Star Wars movies which keep you sitting on the sofa, these exercises will focus on a whole host of muscles, strengthening your hamstrings, calves, and glutes.

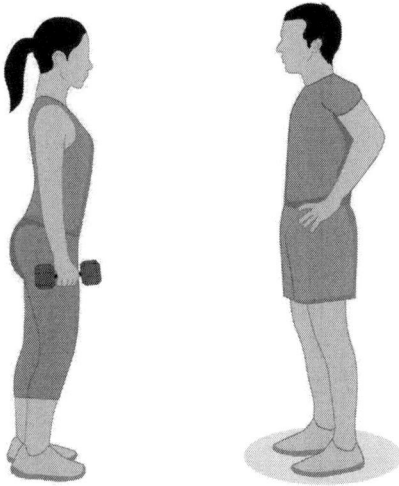

LET'S GRAB SOME WEIGHTS!

#1 – Weighted Glute Bridge

This is the ultimate exercise with many benefits, including reduced back and knee pain, improved posture, and improved sporting activity capacity.

- Lie flat on your back on your exercise mat, bend your knees and keep your feet flat on the ground.
- Place a dumbbell on your stomach, in line with your hips, and hold in position with your hands.
- Push upwards with your feet, pointing your hips towards the ceiling and squeezing your glutes simultaneously.
- Form a straight line with your knees, hips, and shoulders.
- Hold for thirty seconds, then slowly relax back onto your exercise mat.
- This is one rep.
- You can start by doing 1 set of 10 reps but by the second week of practicing, you should aim to do 2 sets of 10 reps.

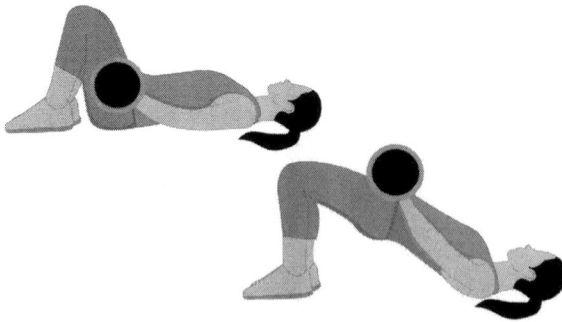

FIGURE 5-1: WEIGHTED GLUTE BRIDGE

#2 – Overhead Shoulder Press

The time has finally arrived to work on your upper body! The overhead shoulder press is excellent for strengthening the whole upper body and will improve your posture and balance.

- Choose two light hand weights. It's best to get the movement right before moving onto heavier weights.
- Stand with your feet apart and a weight in each hand. This should be a comfortable stance; your feet should not be more than shoulder-width apart.
- Hold the weights in front of your shoulders with your palms facing outwards.
- Brace your core and, at the same time, push both weights up towards the ceiling until above your head, extending your arms slowly as you push upwards.
- Bring the weights back to their original position in front of your shoulders.
- Note this should be a slow controlled movement.
- Aim for 3 sets of 10 reps.

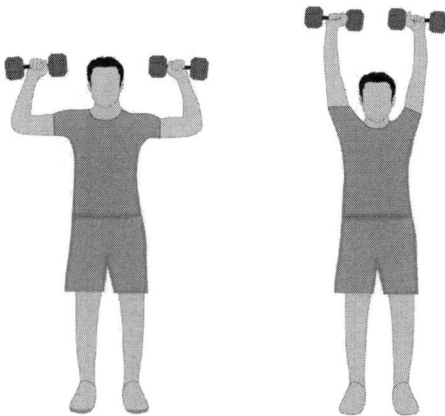

FIGURE 5-2: OVERHEAD SHOULDER PRESS

#3 – Floor Press

The floor press is also known as the chest press for beginners as it helps build strength and better control for heavier weight lifting. This move also prevents unnecessary shoulder stress and reduces the risks of aches and pains.

- Select two light hand weights to start as you will gradually increase the weight as you get stronger.
- Lie on your back with your knees bent and feet flat on the ground.
- With a weight in each hand, keep your upper arms at a forty-five-degree angle to your body. Keep the weights raised in the air.
- Push both weights up simultaneously, extending your arms fully in front of you.
- Fully extend your arms, hold the position for five seconds, and then relax into the original starting position. Remember, this is a slow controlled movement.
- Perform 2 sets of 10 reps.

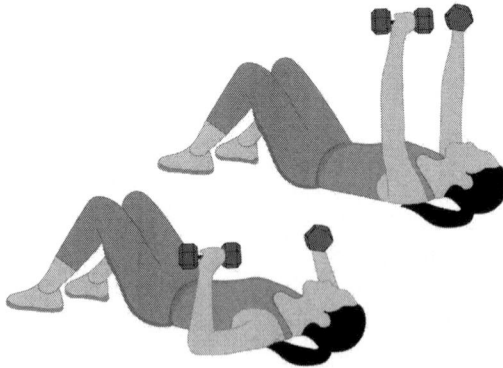

FIGURE 5-3: FLOOR PRESS

#4 – Narrow Row

This is a muscle-building exercise of note, and we strongly recommend that all 50+ers who want to build and maintain strength in their back and shoulders do this one often. Carrying grocery bags, reaching things on a high shelf, carrying a chair – all of these become easy tasks with strong shoulders and back.

- While standing, position your feet shoulder-width apart. Hold a weight in each hand.
- Bend at the waist, maintain a forty-five-degree angle.
- Keep your arms extended, slightly bent at the elbow, and palms facing inwards.
- Tighten your core and pull your arms up, so the hand weights are level with your ribcage; hold for a few seconds and then release.
- Extend your arms back to the original position. Keep your movements slow and controlled.
- You should aim to complete 3 sets of 10 reps.
- Increase reps as your strength increases.

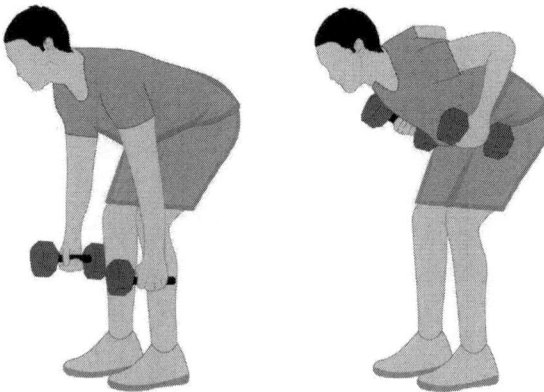

FIGURE 5-4: NARROW ROW

#5 – Weighted Deadlift

This move is slightly more advanced and strengthens the lower back. Incorporating lower back strengthening exercises helps prevent nagging lower back pain, often felt as we get older. If you have back pain or want to avoid ever getting it, this is the exercise for you!

- Stand with your feet shoulder-width apart, knees slightly bent,
- Hold a weight in each hand in front of your thighs, palms facing inwards.
- Keep your core muscles tight and your back flat.
- Bend at the waist, pushing your buttocks out.
- Slowly lower your upper body until the weights pass below your knees.
- Push your hips forward and stand straight up into the original position
- Aim to do 4 sets of 6 reps.
- Look to gradually increase the number of reps.

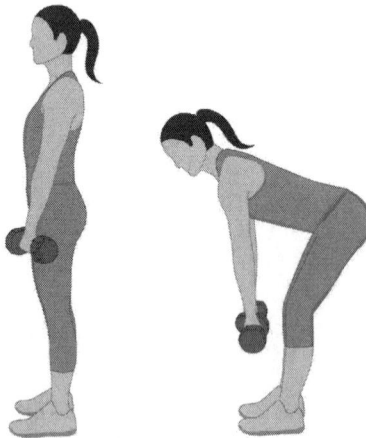

FIGURE 5-5: WEIGHTED DEADLIFT

#6 – **Lat Pullover**

This is an excellent workout for your chest and back muscles. Having a strong back and chest muscles makes everyday reaching, lifting, carrying, and stretching a lot easier.

- Lie on your back, with your knees bent and feet flat on the floor.
- To maintain your balance keep your feet shoulder-width apart.
- Hold the hand weights over your chest, palms facing each other.
- Keep your elbows slightly bent and lower the weights towards the floor above your head.
- Keeping your arms extended and elbows slightly bent, raise the weights until they are above your chest.
- Hold for a few seconds, then lower the weights back onto the floor above your head.
- This movement needs to be slow and controlled.
- Do 3 sets of 8 reps.

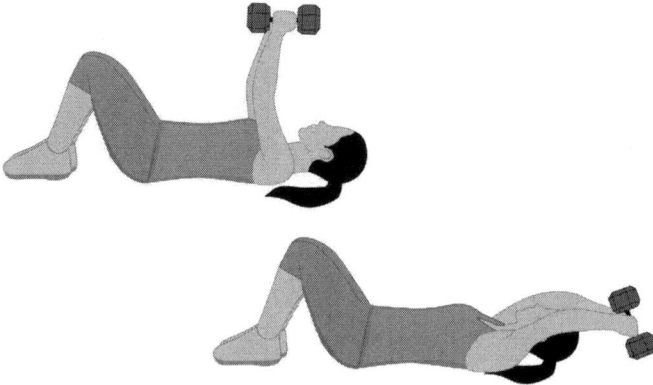

FIGURE 5-6: LAT PULLOVER

#7 – **Floor Chest Flyes**

The floor chest fly is one of our favorites as it's really effective. The strengthening and opening of the chest muscles can reduce upper back pain and increase your upper-body mobility (something we all want!)

- Lie on your back with your knees bent and your feet flat on the floor.
- Holding a weight in each hand, extend your arms out away from the trunk of your body with your palms facing upwards. Visualize your body in the shape of the letter T.
- Lift the weights towards the center of your chest using your chest muscles.
- Touch the weights in the middle, hold this pose and then relax slowly back into the starting position.
- Remember to tighten your abs and keep your elbows slightly bent when lifting to carry out a strong movement.
- Do 3 sets of 10 reps.

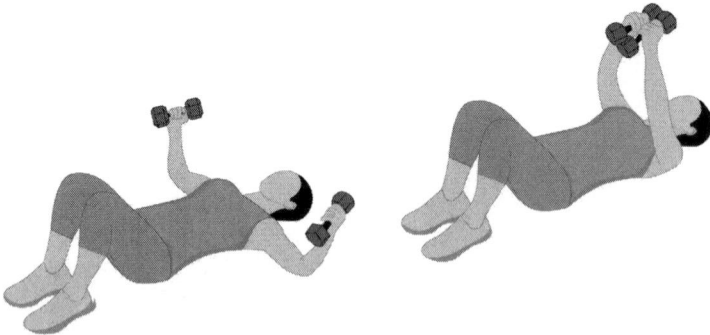

FIGURE 5-7: FLOOR CHEST FLYES

RESISTANCE BANDS

Resistance bands are great for enhancing a host of exercises and movements, which is excellent news for those getting back into fitness after a few years of minimal activity. Take a look at some of these straightforward exercises and try them out for yourself.

#1 – Core Kick

Core kicks are fabulous for toning legs and tightening your core.

- Lie on a mat with your legs extended straight out.
- Bending your right knee, wrap a resistance band around your right foot, holding the ends with both hands.
- Slowly raise that same leg with the resistance band attached bringing your knee up. Keep your core tight.
- Pull your raised knee towards your chest and then slowly push outwards, like a forward kick in slow motion.
- Hold for a few seconds, then slowly return knee to your chest.
- Alternate with the other leg.
- Aim for 3 sets of 6 reps each side.

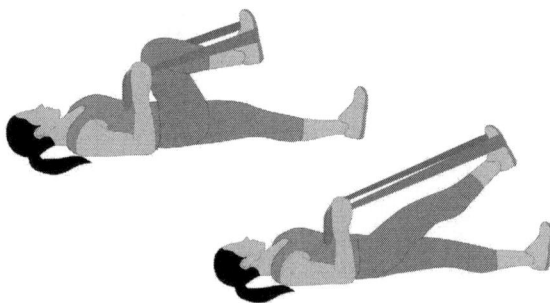

FIGURE 6-1: CORE KICK

#2 – One Arm Tricep Extensions

Tricep extensions are important for joint health. Your triceps are essential for extending your elbow and assisting with extending the shoulders. When you do a tricep extension, you strengthen all the ligaments, tendons, and joints involved in those movements.

- Place your right foot's heel onto the resistance band.
- Pull the band up behind your head with your right hand.
- The band should now be running up the length of your back.
- Extend that same arm entirely above your head and pause.
- Release back into the original position and repeat. That's one rep.
- This movement should not be fast and bouncy; it needs to be slow and steady. Your arm needs to fully extend above your head to gain maximum benefit from this exercise.
- Repeat 2 sets of 8 reps - each side.

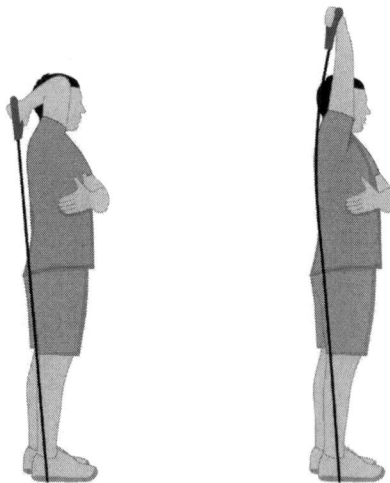

FIGURE 6-2: ONE ARM TRICEP EXTENSIONS

#3 – Resistance Band Bicep Curl

Bicep curls are essential for building muscle mass and increasing strength.

- Place both feet on the mid-section of a resistance band.
- Hold one end in each hand with your arms extended at your sides.
- Pull your hands up, keeping your elbows close to your sides as you squeeze your biceps.
- Your upper body should lean slightly forward to aid with balance, keep your back straight.
- Slowly lower your hands and extend your arms fully at your sides again. This is one rep.
- Repeat 3 sets of 12 reps.

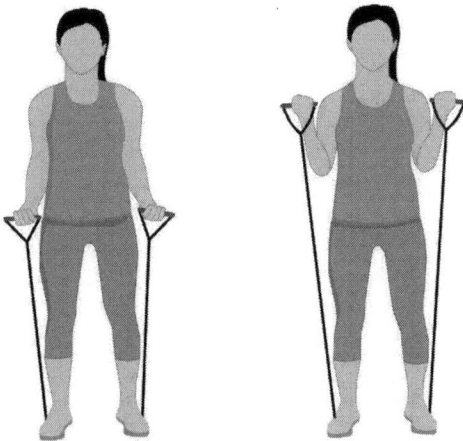

FIGURE 6-3: RESISTANCE BAND BICEP CURL

#4 – Resistance Band Good Morning

This low-impact move is super for beginners and can also be used to warm up the glutes and hamstrings before moving on to more advanced exercises.

- Stand with both feet firmly on one resistance band, keeping your feet comfortably apart, don't over-extend.
- Hold the ends of the band in each hand and keep your arms close to your sides with palms facing inwards.
- Your knees should be slightly bent, don't lock them or make them stiff.
- Bend slowly forward at the hips, pushing your butt out until your upper body is almost parallel to the ground. For this movement, imagine an exaggerated bow.
- Now push your hips up and forward as you straighten back into the original starting position. This is one rep.
- Repeat 2 sets of 12 reps.

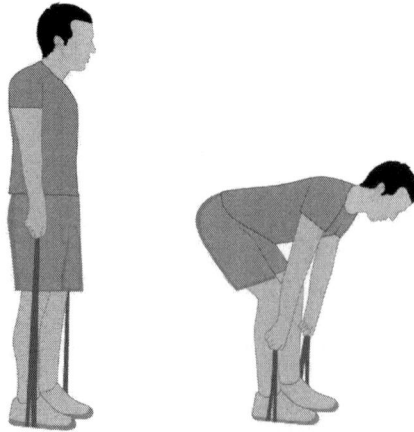

FIGURE 6-4: RESISTANCE BAND GOOD MORNING

#5 – Resistance Band Glute Bridge

This exercise strengthens the thighs, glutes, and core.

- Sitting on an exercise mat, slide a resistance band up and over your knees. The band should sit just above your knees.
- Now lie face up, keeping your knees bent and feet flat on the floor. Your arms should rest at your sides. This is your starting position.
- Tightly squeeze your abs and buttocks as you use your heels to lift your hips up and off the floor. Use your knees to keep tension on the band, so they don't collapse inwards.
- When you lift up, try to make a straight line from your shoulders to your knees and hold this for a few seconds.
- Gently lower your hips back to the floor. This is one rep.
- You can start by doing one set of eight reps.
- Work your way up to 3 sets of 12 reps.

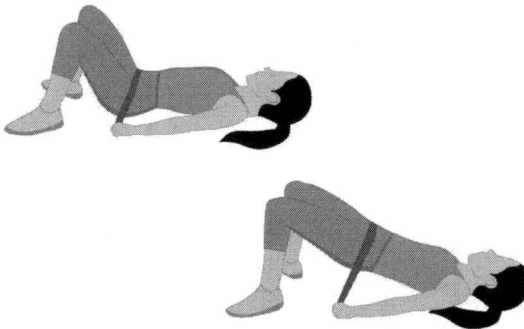

FIGURE 6-5: RESISTANCE BAND GLUTE BRIDGE

#6 – Resistance Band Lateral Walk

We love this exercise because it reminds us of a mini dance routine! It's great for warming up, burning fat, and building strength in your glutes (buttocks) and hips.

- Position your resistance band around your ankles with your knees slightly bent. A gentle squat position is best for this exercise.
- Take a large step to the right with your right foot, then use your left foot to step to the right. Then, place your feet together. Repeat the sequence for five steps.
- Now step to the left with your left foot and follow with your right foot. Repeat the sequence for five steps until you are back at your starting point. This is one rep.
- Continue this step routine, shifting your direction each time.
- At first, it will feel strange, so try to do just two.
- As you get more attuned to the exercise, aim to complete 2 sets of 10 reps.

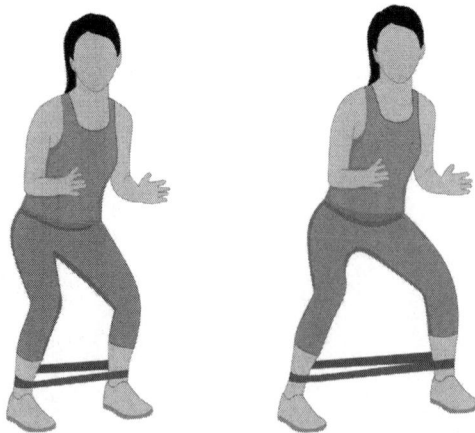

FIGURE 6-6: RESISTANCE BAND LATERAL WALK

#7 – **Resistance Band Pull-Apart**

This reasonably simple move packs a solid punch, enhancing your shoulder strength, mobility, and stability.

- Place your feet hip-width apart, holding a resistance band with both hands.
- Raise the band, so it is at shoulder height in front of you.
- Grip the band tightly, ensuring there is about a foot of resistance band between your hands.
- With a slow controlled movement, pull the band apart so that your hands move outwards to your sides.
- Remember to keep your hands at shoulder height.
- Slowly release the tension and bring your hands back to the starting position. This is one rep.
- Aim to complete 2 sets of 15 reps.

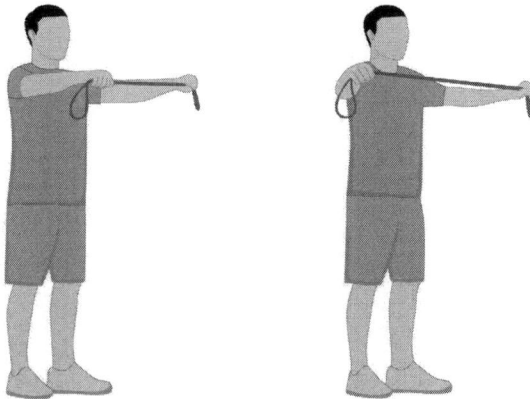

FIGURE 6-7: RESISTANCE BAND PULL-APART

Now that you've got the slightly more complicated yet still oh-so-basic equipment-focused exercises mastered, it's time to move on to our next section, which is all about working out at the gym.

Learn more about the equipment you will find in the gym and how to carry out basic exercises that pack the most punch. Page over to Chapter Seven: *Strength Training at the Gym*

7

STRENGTH TRAINING AT THE GYM

Honestly, there is never a good time to join the gym, is there. We spend our lives making excuses about convenience and tomorrow being a better day. And then suddenly, we're hauling our overweight and untoned bodies over the border of 50, and we realize we never really found the time to go to the gym. We're living proof that tomorrow never comes. The excuse of having kids suddenly becomes having grandkids, and being busy with work suddenly becomes being busy with home maintenance. It's just the way it goes.

But as you get older, the draw of the gym should get stronger. Not because you suddenly wake up with the burning desire to finally get that beach body you spent your youth dreaming about because it's more necessary now than ever before to get fit and active. Working out at home is difficult for some people because there's a lack of motivation (the couch and TV are always just a few steps away). Also, the idea of actually investing in gym equipment is overwhelming. The gym itself, however, is an enticing prospect. It has everything you need for a workout. Professional trainers are nearby to provide advice and help you if you have an exercise-related accident. It also gives you somewhere to go to get out of the house – this alone can motivate some 50+ers.

Joining the gym is a significant step in the right direction. It's not easy to walk into the gym these days with the confidence we once had as twenty-year-olds. Gyms can be viewed as hives of activity filled with youngsters whose toned and fit bodies don't resemble anything that requires the help of a gym membership but don't let this put you off.

The gym machines may seem like you need a three-year university degree to operate them, but they soon become simple devices there for your enjoyment when you understand how to use them.

To swiftly eliminate the confusion from the process, we've compiled a list of gym machines, their uses, and how to use them effectively. After going through each of these explanations and referring to the images, you can operate gym machinery like you're a veritable expert in all things gym-related. All you need to bring is your towel, water bottle, and a dash of confidence. In the words of an unknown author: 'Healthy is an outfit that looks different on everybody,' so forget about how you might appear. Just show up and do the work – you won't regret it.

STRENGTH TRAINING WITH FREE WEIGHTS

This is strength training with resistance exercises using equipment that can be moved around. Some examples are dumbbells, kettlebells, sandbags, and barbells. This section will focus on how this type of training can benefit the whole body while giving you specific guidelines on how to use the equipment to enhance your workout without hurting yourself or becoming a crumpled mess on the floor.

For ease of reference, each body part has been assigned a section detailing the relevant exercises.

CHEST
LEGS & HIPS
BACK & SHOULDERS
ARMS
ABDOMINALS

CHEST

#1 – **Barbell Bench Press**

This exercise builds the chest muscles, triceps, and deltoid shoulder muscles.

- Lie flat on your back on the bench with your feet firmly on the ground positioned below your knees.
- Position your hands slightly wider than shoulder-width.
- Grip the bar tightly and inhale while slowly bringing the bar down to just above your chest.
- Push the bar upwards as you exhale. Remember to focus on a point on the ceiling as you push upwards; this will ensure the bar travels in a straight line each time.
- It's essential to keep your head, shoulders, and hips flat on the bench throughout the lift, creating a firm foundation.
- Use a spotter if you are new to lifting weights.
- Repeat 2 sets of 8 reps, to begin with, but as you get stronger, aim to do 3 sets of 10 reps.

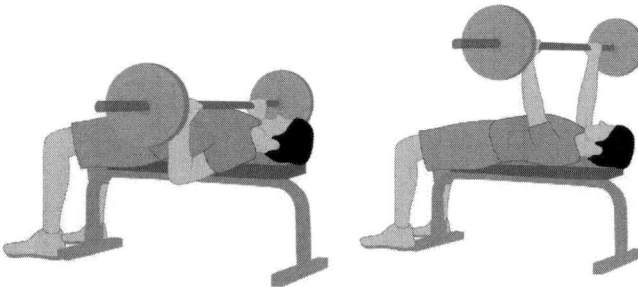

FIGURE 7-1: BARBELL BENCH PRESS

#2 – Incline Barbell Bench Press

With the incline bench press, the bench is positioned at a forty-five-degree angle. This angle creates more focus on the upper chest and front side of your shoulders than a standard bench press would.

- Lie flat on an incline bench; place your hands on the bar shoulder-width apart.
- Keep your shoulder blades firm by pinching them together and driving them into the bench.
- Inhale and lift the bar slowly off the rack. Use a spotter to help you lift off the rack so you can maintain your back's tautness.
- Pause while your back adjusts to the weight, keeping your upper back firm.
- Breathe in deeply as you lower the bar slowly towards your chest.
- Exhale as you push the bar back up towards the rack, press yourself into the bench, pushing down hard with your feet and extending the elbows.
- The bar should touch your chest with each repetition.
- Repeat 2 sets of 8 reps, to begin with, but as you get stronger, aim to do 3 sets of 10 reps.

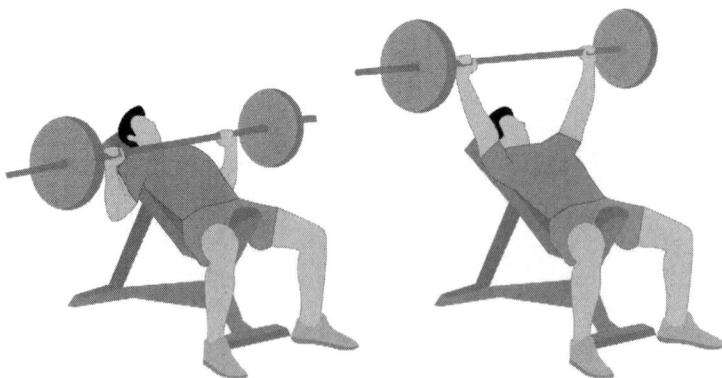

FIGURE 7-2: INCLINE BARBELL BENCH PRESS

#3 – Decline Barbell Bench Press

The bench is set at a fifteen to thirty-degree angle on the decline, meaning your head will be lower than your knees when you are lying on the bench. This design creates more focus on the lower pectorals as you push weights away from your body.

- Lie flat on the decline bench, place your hands on the bar shoulder-width apart, and hook your feet beneath the footpad.
- Put your shoulders firmly back, ensuring the shoulder blades are pinched tightly together and pressed tightly against the bench.
- Inhale and lift the bar slowly off the rack. Use a spotter to help you lift the bar off the rack so you can maintain the tautness in your back.
- Pause while your back adjusts to the weight, keeping your upper back firm.
- Breathe in deeply as you lower the bar slowly towards your chest.
- Exhale as you push the bar back up towards the rack, press yourself into the bench, and extend your elbows.
- Repeat 2 sets of 8 reps, to begin with, but as you get stronger, aim to do 3 sets of 10 reps.

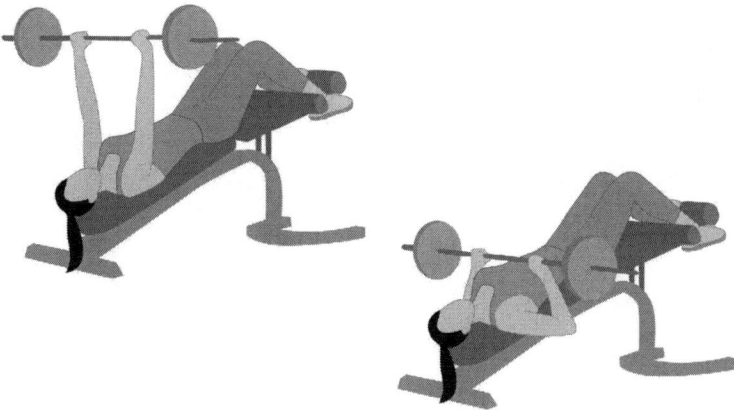

FIGURE 7-3 : DECLINE BARBELL BENCH PRESS

#4 – Dumbbell Flat Bench Flyes

This exercise works the tops of the shoulders and the pectoral muscle of your chest. It also helps to strengthen the upper back and biceps. Sit on a bench with legs on either side and feet on the floor.

- Hold a dumbbell in each hand, rest them on your thighs with the palms of your hands facing inwards.
- Slowly lower your upper body until you lie flat on the bench with the dumbbells close to your chest.
- Raise the dumbbells above your chest, hands together.
- Keeping your arms slightly bent, open up your arms lowering the dumbbells until they are on either side of you. The dumbbells should be level with your chest on both sides.
- Using a slow controlled motion, close your arms, returning the dumbbells to the starting position above your chest. Remember to squeeze your pecs together at the same time.
- To begin with, repeat 2 sets of 8 reps. As you get stronger, aim to do 3 sets of 10 reps.
- *Tip: Heavyweights are not required for this exercise. Use your chest muscles and not your arms when lifting.

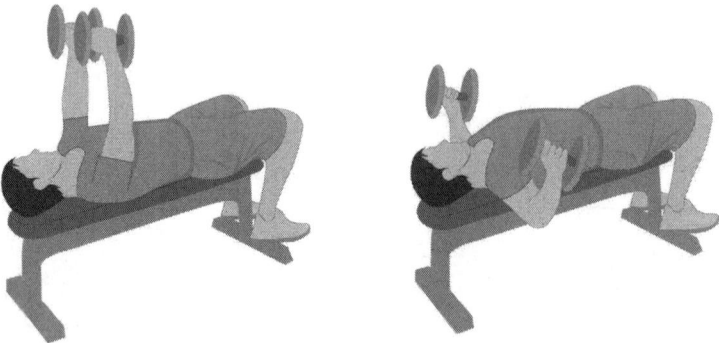

FIGURE 7-4: DUMBBELL FLAT BENCH FLYES

LEGS & HIPS

Legs and hips are often the last on the list when it comes to muscle strengthening. Just like breathing, our legs and hips continue to function without us giving them much thought. However, strengthening the muscles in your hips and legs improves stability and flexibility, ensuring you can move easily and avoid injuries.

Hip weakness and stiffness can be attributed to excessive sitting and no exercise, which would explain a lot for those of us stuck behind a desk every day of the week or just sitting around the house all day.

IT'S LEG DAY!

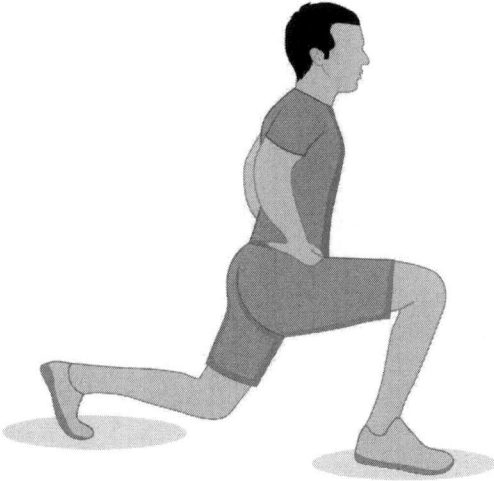

#1 – Barbell Squats

This exercise directly strengthens your hamstrings, glutes, and groin muscles. Strengthening these muscles promotes flexibility and balance.

- Place a bar in the rack; this should be positioned just below shoulder height, then select the weight plates you wish to use. Beginners should choose lighter-weight plates while learning how to execute this exercise.
- Place your hands slightly more than shoulder-width apart.
- Step under the bar and rest the barbell on your back.
- Push up with your legs, lift the bar off the rack; take a step back from the rack. Remember to keep your feet shoulder-width apart and your knees slightly bent.
- Keep your core tight and your head and spine in line.
- Start the squat by bending at the knees, hips, and lower body. Remember to keep your heels flat on the floor.
- Now push up out of the squat into the starting position, using your legs as the driving force.
- Do 2 sets of 8 reps (as you get stronger, do 3 sets of 10 reps).

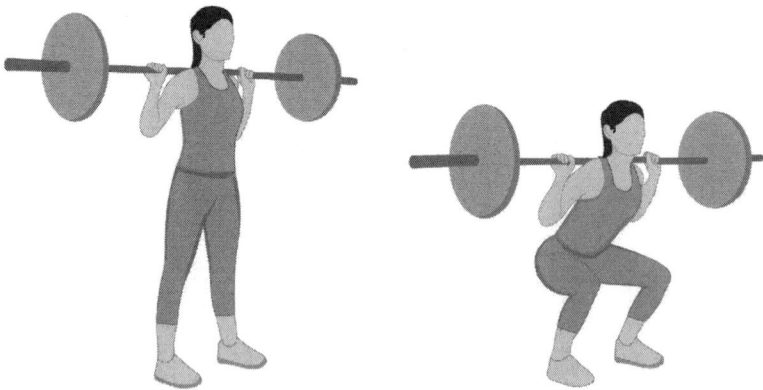

FIGURE 8-1: BARBELL SQUATS

#2 – Freestanding Modified Lunge

Lunges are great for building strength and toning your body. They work a range of muscles, including the abdominals, back muscles, glutes, hamstrings, and calves. In addition, lunges strengthen your core, buttocks, and legs.

- Place a barbell on the rack, just below shoulder height.
- Step under the bar with your shoulders positioned under it. Be sure the bar is resting on your shoulders and not your neck.
- Place your hands on the bar using an overhand grip with your elbows at a ninety-degree angle.
- Lift the barbell off the rack and step away from the rack.
- Using your left foot, step forward and squat down slowly, keeping your back straight.
- Lower your body until your right knee almost touches the floor.
- Push up out of the lunge using your left heel as the driving force. Exhale as you move up out of the lunge.
- Repeat 2 sets of 10 reps - on each side.

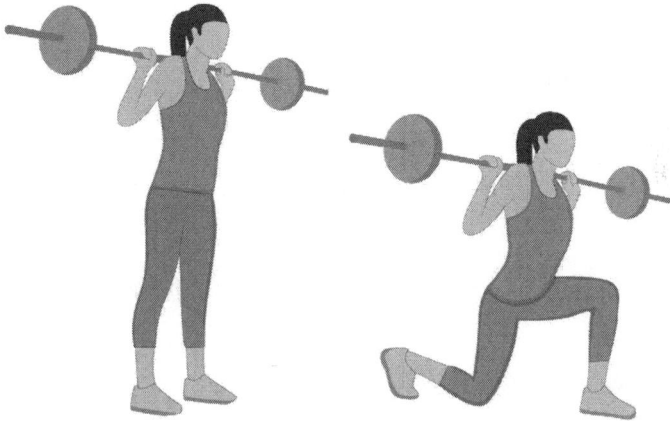

FIGURE 8-2: FREESTANDING MODIFIED LUNGE

BACK & SHOULDERS

Strong shoulders make everyday lifting easier and safer, while a strong back prevents back pain and promotes better posture. In addition, strength training of the upper back can help with back pain suffered by desk-bound professionals.

#1 – Bent Over One-Arm Dumbbell Rows

This exercise strengthens the forearm and bicep muscles, upper back muscles as well as your grip.

- Place a dumbbell on the floor next to the weight bench.
- Standing side-on to the bench, place your left knee and left palm on the seat.
- Keeping your back straight, bend forward until your back is parallel to the floor, and with your right hand, pick up the dumbbell, keeping your core tight.
- Holding the dumbbell start the row. Squeeze your lat muscles while keeping your arm close to your body.
- Push your elbow up towards the ceiling. The dumbbell should touch your lower chest during this movement, and your elbow should not go higher than your back.
- Lower the dumbbell back towards the floor.
- Repeat 2 sets of 8 reps, then do the other arm.

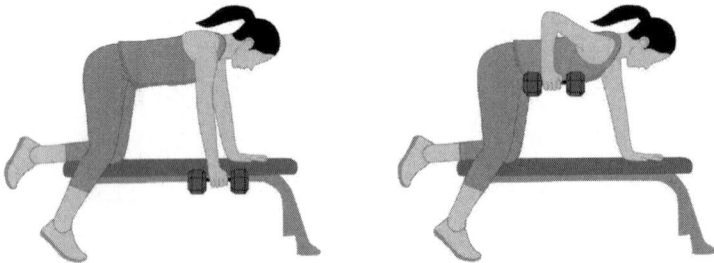

FIGURE 9-1: BENT OVER ONE-ARM DUMBBELL ROWS

#2 – Barbell Seated Front Shoulder Press

This exercise increases strength in the Deltoid muscles, improves balance, and helps achieve a toned look.

- After bringing up the barbell to your chest and shoulders, sit on an adjustable bench with your knees apart and feet flat on the floor.
- Your hands should be placed on the bar a little wider than shoulder-width.
- Keep your core tight and your elbows tucked in.
- Exhale as you push the barbell up towards the ceiling, extending your arms fully above your shoulders.
- Inhale as you slowly lower the barbell to the just in front of your shoulders.
- Repeat 2 sets of 8 reps to begin.
- As you get stronger, aim to do 4 sets of 10 reps.

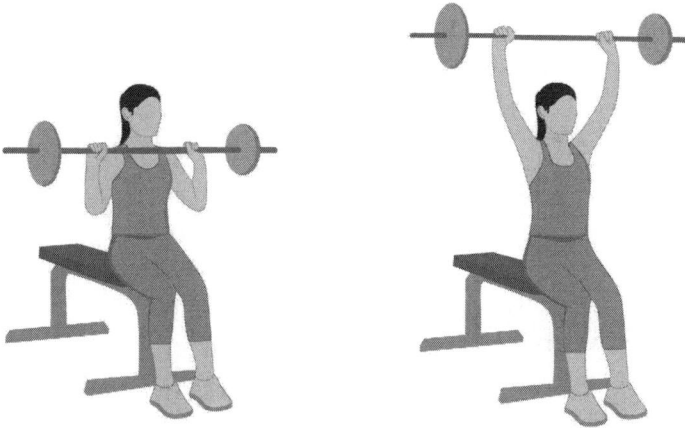

FIGURE 9-2: BARBELL SEATED FRONT SHOULDER PRESS

#3 – Barbell Press Behind Neck

This exercise is used to improve upper back and shoulder strength.

- Select the weight plates you wish to use; beginners should opt for lighter weights until they are confident with the lift.
- Sit on the bench with your feet placed flat on the ground and spaced slightly wider than shoulder-width.
- Place your hands on the bar, knuckles up, and thumb wrapped around the bar then unrack the bar.
- Inhale deeply, brace your body and tuck your chin into your chest.
- Slowly lower the bar to the back of your neck. Don't place the bar on your neck; it should be held just above this area.
- Exhale and slowly push the bar upwards until your arms are fully extended.
- Repeat 2 sets of 8 reps to begin with, but as you get stronger, aim to do 3 sets of 10 reps.
- *TIP: This is an advanced exercise that is best done with a spotter assisting.

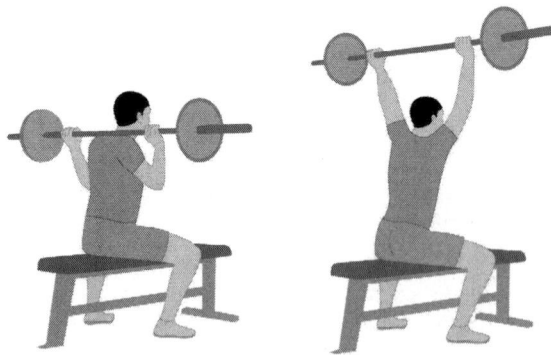

FIGURE 9-3: BARBELL PRESS BEHIND NECK

#4 – Upright Rows

This exercise is used to develop the rhomboid, trapeze, and bicep muscles.

- Place a barbell on the floor in front of you. Select weight plates until you are confident with the lift.
- Position your feet a comfortable distance apart
- Pick the barbell up with arms fully extended, allow the barbell to hang freely in front of your thighs, palms facing inwards. Your hands should be shoulder-width apart.
- Inhale, keeping your core tight, back straight, and chest up.
- Slowly bring the barbell upwards to chin level; your elbows should be pointing up and outwards. Exhale during this movement. Your arms go no higher than your shoulders.
- Pause for a second with the barbell at chin level, then slowly lower the bar to the starting position, inhaling as you release.
- Keep your legs straight throughout the lift.
- Repeat 2 sets of 8 reps, but as you get stronger, aim to do 3 sets of 10 reps.

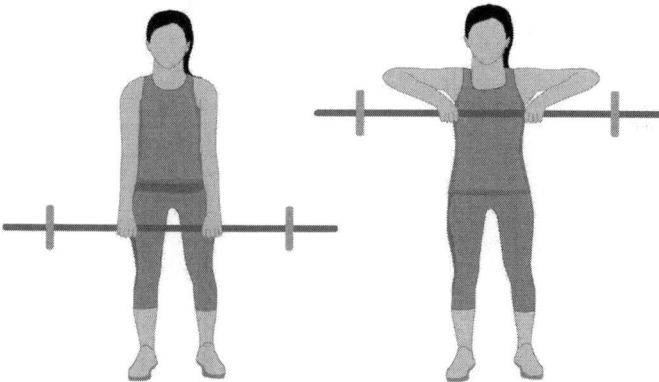

FIGURE 9-4: UPRIGHT ROWS

#5 – Dumbbells Standing Lateral Raise

This exercise can aid with increasing shoulder size and improved shoulder mobility. In addition, your core and muscles in the upper back, arms, and neck all receive a thorough workout with this lift.

- Standing with your feet comfortably apart, hold a dumbbell in each hand with palms facing inwards.
- Keep your back and legs straight with the dumbbells held slightly away from the sides of your body. This keeps the tension in the deltoids on your sides.
- Slowly raise your arms outwards; your body should resemble a star shape. The dumbbells should go no higher than shoulder height.
- Pause, then slowly lower the dumbbells to the starting position.
- When lowering the dumbbells, ensure they don't touch your body.
- Repeat 2 sets of 8 reps, to begin with, but as you get stronger, aim to do 3 sets of 10 reps.

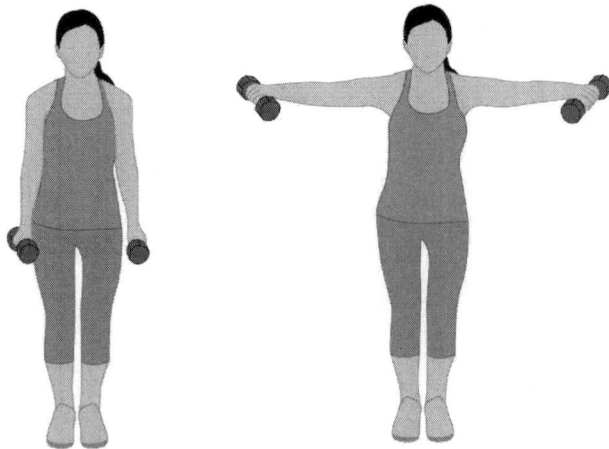

FIGURE 9-5: DUMBBELLS STANDING LATERAL RAISE

#6 – Dumbbell Standing Front Raise

This lift is perfect for beginners and can also be helpful if you are recovering from a shoulder injury. As humans, we need strong shoulders for everyday lifting activities, not just when pressing weights at the gym. This lift works the deltoids and pectoral muscles and builds strength and definition in the fronts and sides of your shoulders.

- Select two lightweight dumbbells.
- Position your feet shoulder-width apart. Keep your arms fully extended down at your sides. Posture is essential here. Keep your back straight and your chest out.
- Grip the dumbbells ensuring your palms are facing inwards.
- Tighten your abdominal muscles and lift the weights upwards, stretching your arms out in front of you. Your palms should be facing downwards as you lift.
- Your elbows should be slightly bent to reduce stress in the joints.
- You should feel the tension in your shoulders.
- Slowly lower your arms and return the dumbbells to the original position at your sides.
- Repeat two 2 of 8 reps to begin with, but as you get stronger, aim to do 3 sets of 10 reps.

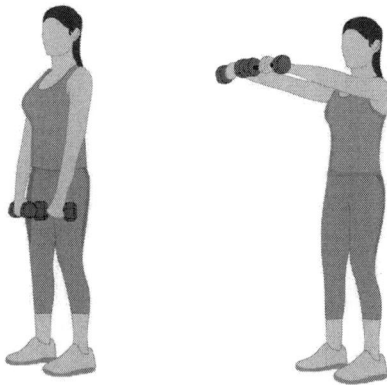

FIGURE 9-6: DUMBBELL STANDING FRONT RAISE

#7 – Dumbbell Shoulder Shrugs

This lift is an excellent way to increase the strength and size of the trapezius muscles. These muscles are found in the upper back and play a significant role in supporting your posture. It also exercises the brachioradialis muscle in your forearm, increasing forearm strength at the same time.

- Place a pair of dumbbells on the floor, stand in between them with your feet spaced comfortably apart.
- Bend from the waist down while tightening your core and grip a dumbbell with each hand. Ensure your palms are facing inwards.
- Raise your upper body into an upright standing position with your back straight and core engaged. The dumbbells should hang at your sides.
- Tighten your traps, bringing your shoulders up and back at the same time.
- Squeeze your traps hard, pause, then slowly lower your shoulders, allowing the dumbbell to return to the original position at your sides.
- Repeat 2 sets of 8 reps to begin with, but as you get stronger, aim to do 3 sets of 10 reps.

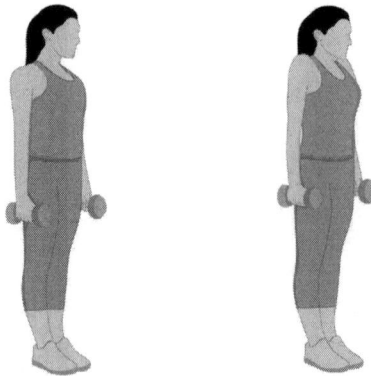

FIGURE 9-7: DUMBBELL SHOULDER SHRUGS

#8 – Rotator Cuff Stabilization Many exercises help with rotator cuff stabilization. These exercises are mostly used to increase strength after suffering a shoulder injury; however, they can also be used to maintain and strengthen the Rotator cuff to prevent injury from occurring. We have selected one exercise to illustrate this technique.

Side-Lying External Rotation

- Lie down on the side opposite to your shoulder injury.
- Bend your injured arm, forming a ninety-degree angle, and prop your elbow on your side. This will provide support.
- Have a light dumbbell resting on the floor in front of you.
- Using your injured arm's hand, grip the dumbbell.
- Keeping your elbow tucked in against your side, slowly raise the dumbbell towards the ceiling. This movement will cause your shoulder to rotate backward and forwards.
- Be careful when raising the dumbbell; make sure your movements are slow and controlled. STOP if any pain or strain is felt as you don't want to cause further injury.
- Hold the dumbbell up for a few seconds with your elbow resting on your side before lowering the dumbbell.
- Repeat 3 sets of 10 reps.

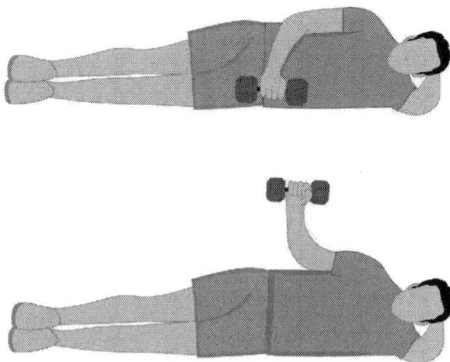

FIGURE 9-8: ROTATOR CUFF STABILATION

ARMS

Some fascinating truths about arm strengthening exercises include
building bone density and improving circulation, reducing the risk of
osteoporosis and heart diseases. In addition, by strengthening your arms,
you are also adding to the strength of your upper body, which aids
posture and balance and boosts endurance in sporting activities.

In the following pages we show you a variety of workouts that you can
schedule into your regular routine.

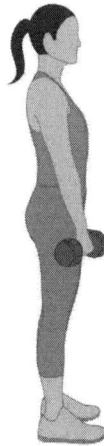

Let's work on those arms!

#1 – Seated Overhead Triceps Extension

- Sit upright on a bench and place your feet firmly on the floor.
- With both hands, hold a dumbbell at one end, palms facing inwards.
- Lift the dumbbell slowly into the air until it is above and behind your head. Your arms should be fully extended.
- Keep your biceps as close to your head as possible.
- Lower the dumbbell behind your head until your forearms and biceps are touching. Hold for one second.
- The dumbbell should be behind your back about mid-shoulder blade height, and your elbows should be pointing towards the ceiling.
- Lift the weight up and back into the start position with your arms fully extended. This movement is completed using the triceps.
- Repeat 2 sets of 8 reps to begin with, but as you get stronger aim to do 3 sets of 10 reps.

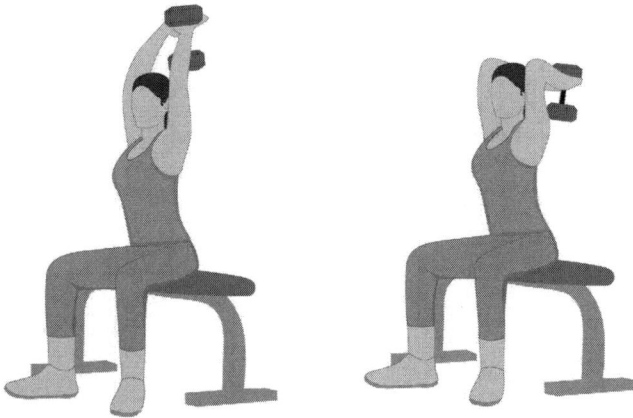

FIGURE 10-1: SEATED OVERHEAD TRICEP EXTENSION

#2 – Supine Barbell French Curl

Also called the triceps extension, this lift helps to build your triceps.

- Lie on a bench keeping your back straight and your core tight.
- Your feet should be flat on the floor.
- Reach up for the bar with your arms fully extended. Using an overhand grip, place your hands at a narrow grip for this lift.
- Keep your core tight and lift the bar off the rack.
- Slowly lower the bar behind your head as low as you can. Remember to keep your elbows tucked close to your head and your back flush with the bench.
- You should feel your triceps stretch as you lower the bar.
- Push the bar back up, straightening your arms until fully extended, and return to the starting position. Only your forearms should be moving during this lift.
- Repeat 2 sets of 8 reps to begin with, but as you get stronger, aim to do 3 sets of 10 reps.

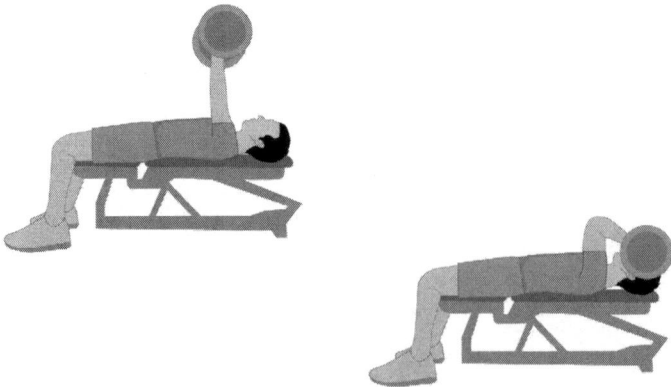

FIGURE 10-2: SUPINE BARBELL FRENCH CURL

#3 – Dumbbell Kickbacks

This is the perfect exercise for full tricep development.

- Standing side-on to the bench, place your left knee and left palm on the seat.
- Keeping your back straight, bend forward until your back is parallel to the floor.
- With your right hand, pick up the dumbbell and hold it at a ninety-degree angle.
- Using a slow, smooth movement, extend your forearm backward while flexing your triceps simultaneously.
- Return to the starting position by bending your arm at a ninety-degree angle.
- Repeat 2 sets of 8 reps to begin with, but as you get stronger, aim to do 3 sets of 10 reps for each side.

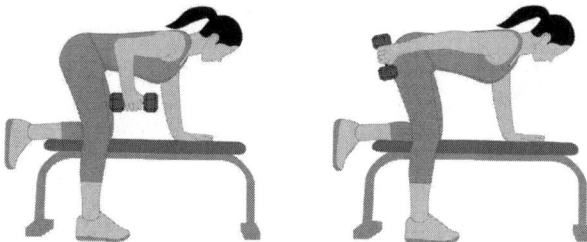

FIGURE 10-3: DUMBBELL KICKBACKS

#4 – Standing Barbell Curl

This lift is an intense workout for the biceps, helping to increase strength.

- Your hands need to be placed shoulder-width apart on the barbell, use an underhand grip with palms facing upwards
- Stand straight up put one foot slightly back for stability.
- Keep your back straight and your arms fully extended out in front of you.
- Ensure your elbows are tucked in closely to your sides.
- Slowly curl the bar upwards towards your collar bone.
- Squeeze your biceps as you curl upwards, then slowly lower the bar to the starting position.
- Repeat 2 sets of 8 reps to begin with, but as you get stronger, aim to do 3 sets of 10 reps.

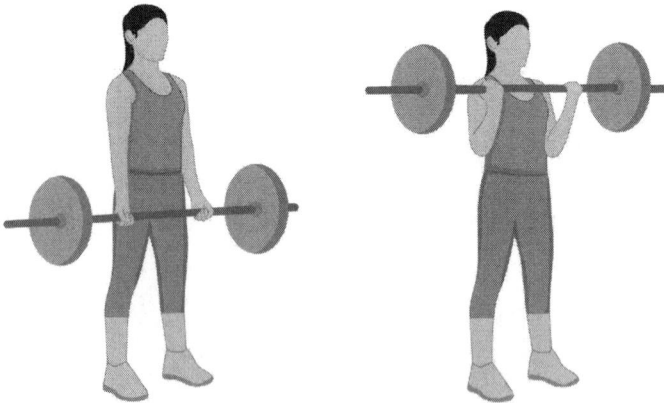

FIGURE 10-4: STANDING BARBELL CURL

#5 – Dumbbell Concentration Curl

This exercise is popular for increasing the strength and size of the bicep.

- Position yourself in a seated position on a gym bench, place your feet firmly on the floor.
- Select a dumbbell that is not too heavy for you.
- Rest the upper arm of the hand, holding the dumbbell against the inner thigh on the same side.
- You may need to open your legs quite wide to do this. Using this support enables the tension to be concentrated in the biceps.
- Keep your back straight and your abdominal muscles tight.
- Slowly curl the dumbbell up towards your chin, keep your upper arm resting on the inner thigh throughout this movement.
- Squeeze the bicep at the top of the curl, then lower the dumbbell slowly back into the starting position.
- Repeat 2 sets of 8 reps to begin with, but as you get stronger, aim to do 3 sets of 10 reps.
- Tip: When lowering your arm, do so slowly, maintaining tension on the bicep the whole way down.

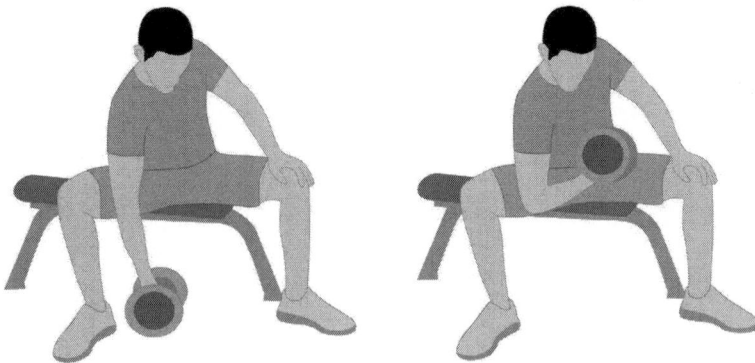

FIGURE 10-5: DUMBBELL CONCENTRATION CURL

#6 – Barbell Wrist Curl

This lift improves forearm strength enabling you to lift heavier weights by strengthening your grip.

- Select suitable weight plates and load them onto the bar.
- Assume a seated position on an upright bench with your feet firmly placed on the floor.
- Rest your forearms on your thighs, using palms up grip called a supinated grip.
- Slowly curl the bar towards you using only your wrists.
- Your forearms should remain on your thighs throughout this movement.
- Slowly lower the bar back into the starting position.
- Repeat 2 sets of 8 reps to begin with, but as you get stronger, aim to do 3 sets of 10 reps.

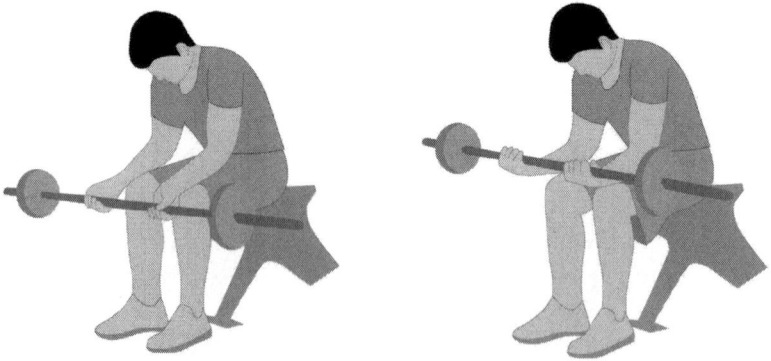

FIGURE 10-6: BARBELL WRIST CURL

ABDOMINALS

Abdominals support the muscles in the mid and lower back. Weak abdominals force the back muscles to work harder to support your middle. Strengthening these muscles improves their strength and endurance preventing fatigue and injury.

#1 – Dumbbell Side Bends

This exercise strengthens the external and internal obliques.

- Stand with your feet shoulder-width apart, your back straight, and your core tight.
- Hold a dumbbell in both hands, palm facing inwards.
- Slowly bend to your right side and pause.
- Feel the stretch.
- Now straighten back up into the original starting position.
- Bend to the left side and pause.
- Complete 30 repetitions (15 on each side).

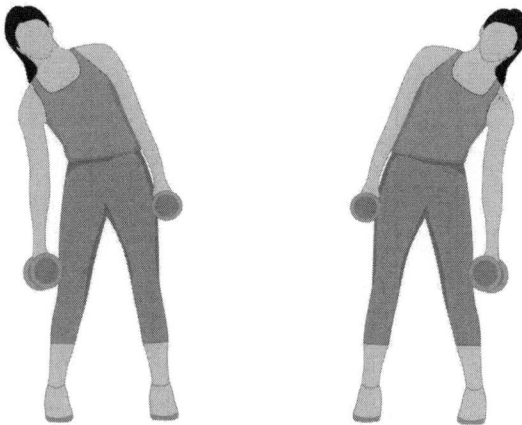

FIGURE 11-1: DUMBBELL SIDE BENDS

EXERCISES USING EQUIPMENT & MACHINES

Learning how to use the gym equipment correctly can take a lot of the guesswork out of exercising. There's a piece of gym equipment to work out every area of your body. How convenient!

In this next chapter is an explanation of each exercise for each body zone, using the equipment. The pictures should help you identify the equipment on the gym floor.

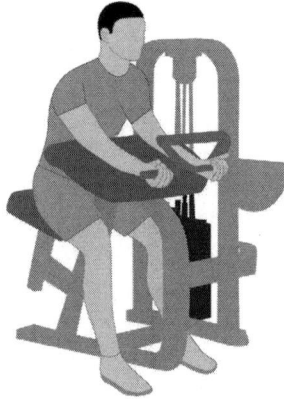

LET'S GET INTO THE GYM!

CHEST

#1 – **Pec Deck Machine**

This exercise increases the strength and muscle mass of your chest. It targets the pectoralis muscles. It's ideal for strengthening your torso and stabilizing your shoulders. Start by choosing a suitable weight for the machine.

- Adjust the seat pad height, so the handles are at chest height.
- Sit up tall and place your feet comfortably on the floor with the back pad supporting your spine.
- Relax your neck and shoulders. Grab the handles with each hand, so your palms are facing forward.
- Press your arms together in front of your chest in a slow controlled movement.
- Pause for a little while and slowly bring your arms back to the starting position. Perform 2 sets of 7 reps.
- Work your way up to 3 sets of 10 reps.
- TIP: Breathe with each movement; exhale as you bring your arms together and inhale as you return to an open position.

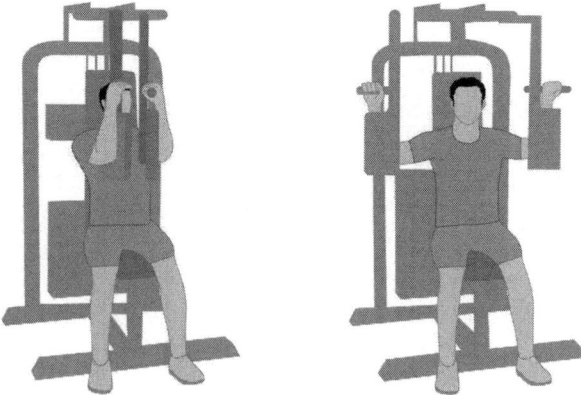

FIGURE 12-1: PEC DECK MACHINE

#2 – Body-Weight Dips

The dip machine exercise strengthens the tricep muscles at the back of your upper arms, the deltoid muscles of your shoulders, and the upper pectoralis muscles of your chest.

- Stand or kneel on the levered platform before adding any weight. Grasp the handles of the machine with straight elbows.
- Test how far you can lower yourself without arching your back or any assistance.
- Once your arms bend to 90 degrees, push yourself back to a straight arm position.
- Move the pin on the machine to the weight plate you need and try again.
- The correct weight should let you lower yourself smoothly and return to the starting position with moderate effort.
- Keep your body centered and the core muscles taut.
- Perform at least 2 sets of 10 reps.

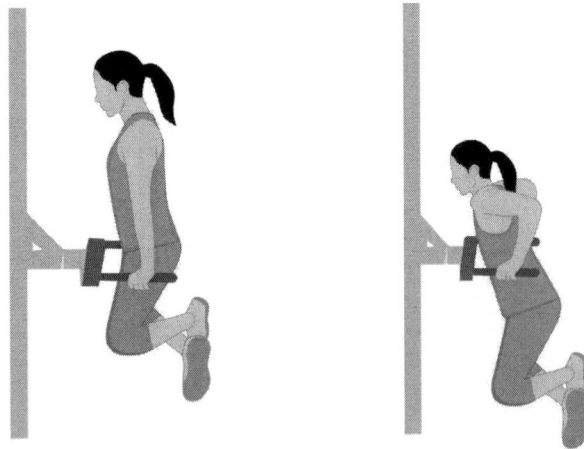

FIGURE 12-2: BODY-WEIGHT DIPS

#3 – Cable Crossover

This exercise strengthens the pectoralis major muscles at the bottom of your chest and activates your shoulder and back muscles. The standing cable crossover recruits the most chest muscle fibers. Start by standing between the two cable stations with the pulley handles on each side.

- Hold the handles with an overhand grip. Your arms should be outstretched.
- Lean forward by bending your knees and hips slightly, but not too far.
- Pull your hands down in front of your body in a hugging motion.
- Keep your elbows in a fixed, bent position as you bring your hands to meet around your mid-section.
- Slowly return to the starting position.
- Inhale when relaxing and exhale when contracting.
- Repeat 3 sets of 10 reps.

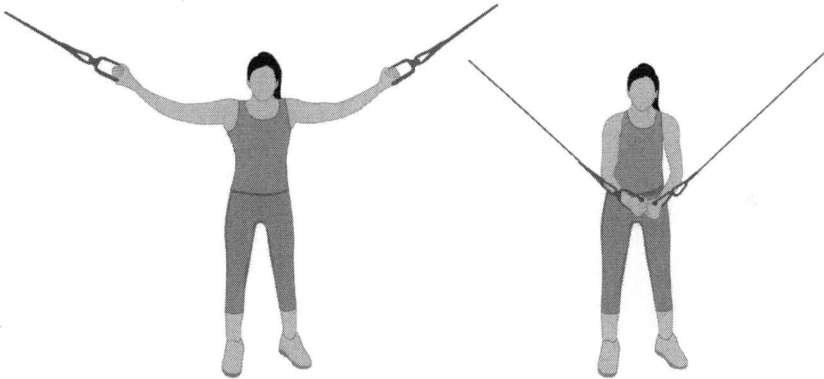

FIGURE 12-3: CABLE CROSSOVER

LEGS & HIPS

#1 – Machine Incline Leg Press

This exercise strengthens the quadriceps of your thighs. It also develops the hamstrings, calves, and gluteus (buttocks) muscles. Sit on the machine and comfortably rest your head and back on the padded support. Place your feet hip wide on the platform and ensure they're flat.

- Release the safety bars, grasp the side handles and extend your legs, so your torso and legs form a 90 degrees angle.
- While bracing your abdominal muscles, push the platform away with your forefoot and heels.
- You should never exclusively use the front of your foot or toes to move the pad forward.
- Now extend your legs and keep your head and back flat against the pad as you exhale. Extend slowly rather than explosively.
- Pause at the top of the movement. Return the footplate to the start position as you inhale by bending your knees gradually.
- Start with 2 sets of 10 leg presses and advance from there as you build strength.

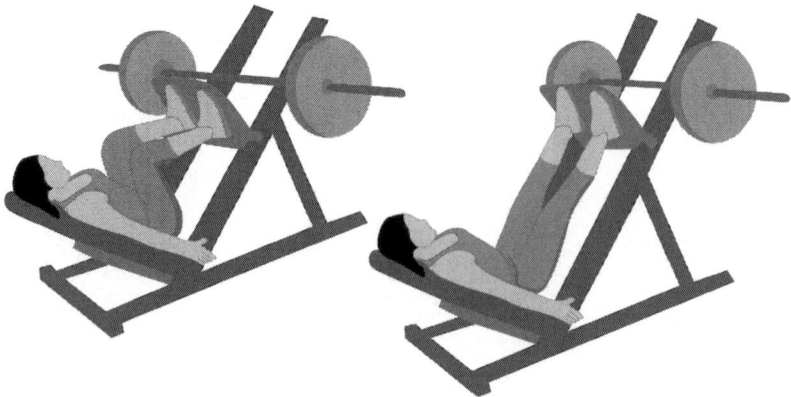

FIGURE 13-1: MACHINE INCLINE LEG PRESS

#2 – Hack Squat Machine

This exercise predominantly strengthens the quads and glutes. It also activates the calves, hamstrings, abdominals, and spinal erectors or back muscles. Start by loading the machine with the desired amount of weight. If you're a beginner, familiarize yourself with the machine movement before adding weight.

- Position yourself in the machine by placing your feet shoulder-width apart.
- Place your shoulders and back against the pads.
- Release the safety handles, inhale and lower the weight slowly by bending your knees until they reach a 90-degree angle.
- Pause a few seconds, then push up through the back of your feet to extend your legs back to the start position.
- Once you can easily complete a few sets, add more weight gradually.
- Do 3 sets of 10 reps.

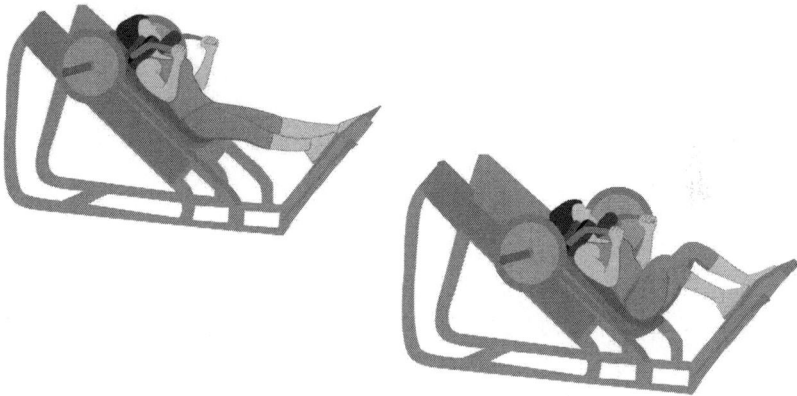

FIGURE 13-2: HACK SQUAT MACHINE

#3 – Cable Hip Extensions

This is an excellent isolation exercise that strengthens and increases the size of your gluteus maximus. It also activates and develops the hamstrings.

- Start by selecting the desired weight.
- Clip a low cable to an ankle strap and attach it securely to your right ankle.
- Stand tall in front of the cable machine with your back upright and core tight.
- Hold on to the cable machine for balance if necessary.
- Exhale and move your right foot up and back while balancing your weight on your left leg until your hip is fully extended.
- Pause at this position for a few seconds, inhale, and bring your foot down slowly to the start position.
- Repeat 2 sets of 10 reps - on each side.

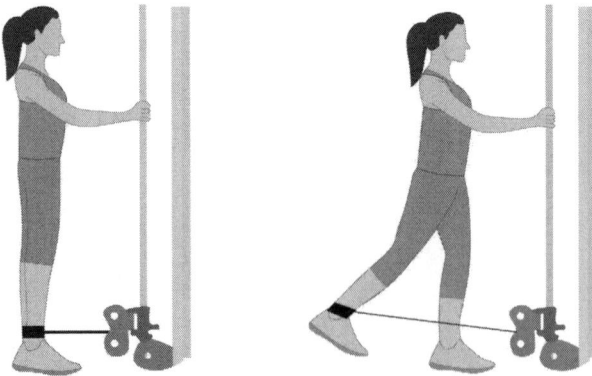

FIGURE 13-3: CABLE HIP EXTENSIONS

#4 – Hip Adductor Machine

This exercise strengthens the hip adductor muscles in your inner thigh and helps build shapely inner thighs. It also helps prevent injury and improves athletic performance.

- Start by selecting the desired weight.
- Bring the pads together so you can sit and place your feet on the footrests.
- Your knees should be outside the knee pads.
- Place your hands on the handles and brace your core.
- Assume a good starting point by moving the pads out as far as comfortably possible.
- You should feel a mild stretch in your inner thighs.
- Maintain an upright position with your back against the pad and spine neutral.
- Exhale and bring your knees back together as you squeeze the pads inward.
- Once the pads touch, return slowly to the start position.
- Repeat 3 sets of 10 reps.

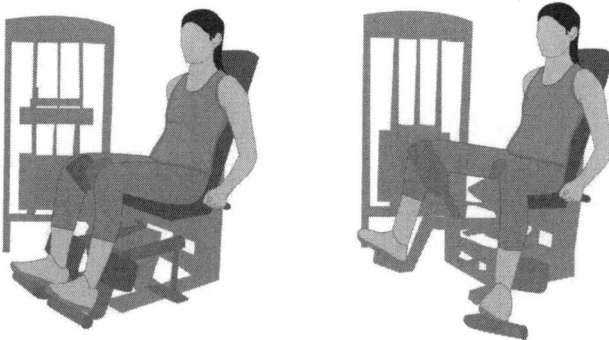

FIGURE 13-4: HIP ADDUCTOR MACHINE

#5 – Hip Abductor Machine

This exercise helps strengthen the hip abductor muscles found in your outer thighs and around your glutes. You'll get a tight and toned backside and prevent hip or knee pain.

- Move the pin to the desired weight.
- Sit on the abductor machine with your feet flat on the footrests and hands on each handle grip.
- Your thighs should be on the inside of the legs pads. This is your starting position, with your knees together.
- Now exhale as you push your legs outwards against the pads, separating them as far as possible.
- Hold this position for a few seconds. Now inhale as you slowly return to the starting position.
- Start with little weight and add more as you perfect your form and gain confidence.
- Repeat 3 sets of 10 reps.

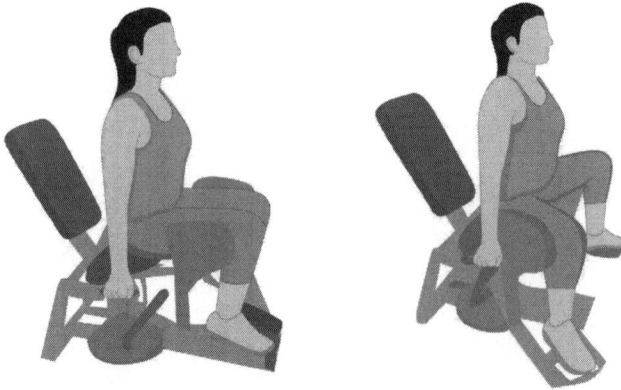

FIGURE 13-5: HIP ABDUCTOR MACHINE

#6 – **Machine Seated leg extension:**

This exercise strengthens the quadriceps muscles at the front of your thigh, including the vastus muscles and the rectus femoris.

- Select a weight with moderate load and sit on the leg extension machine. Place your legs under the pad with feet pointed forward.
- The pad should be at the top of your legs at the ankles and your knees at 90 degrees.
- Firmly grip the hand bars. This is your start position.
- Exhale and lift the weight by extending your legs until they're almost straight.
- Hold for a few seconds and lower the weight slowly to the start position.
- Keep your back straight on the backrest and don't lock your knees or arch your back.
- Repeat 3 sets of 10 reps.

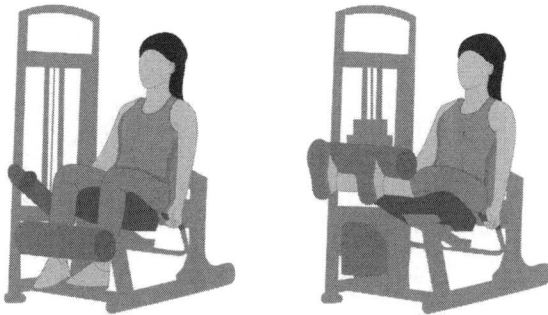

FIGURE 13-6: MACHINE SEATED LEG EXTENSION

#7 – Machine Lying Leg Curl

This exercise improves the strength and flexibility of your hamstrings. It also works on your gluteus muscles (buttocks), thighs, and the shins' front (tibialis anterior).

- Start by lying flat on your stomach.
- Adjust the roller pad, so it rests comfortably right under your calves above the heels. Ensure the pads aren't too high up, as this can reduce your range of motion.
- Fully stretch out your legs. Now inhale and lightly grasp the handles.
- Smoothly lift your feet as you exhale, keep your hips firmly on the bench, and pull your ankles as close to your buttocks as you can.
- Pause and maintain focus as you prepare to lower your legs.
- Inhale and return your feet to the starting position in a slow, smooth, controlled movement.
- Repeat 3 sets of 10-12 reps.
- TIP: You can use your toes to target the calf muscles and hamstrings by curling them or pointing them out.

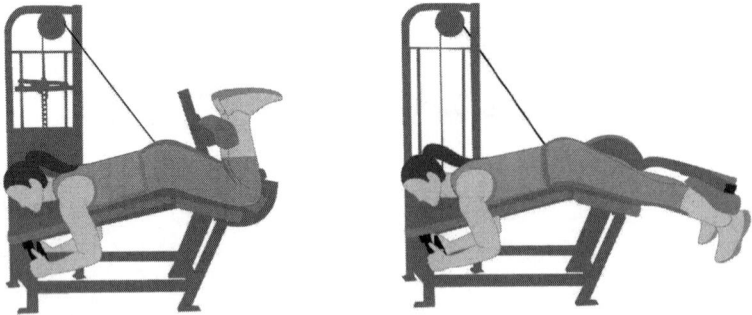

FIGURE 13-7: MACHINE LYING LEG CURL

#8 – Machine Seated Calf Raise

You can use this exercise to increase the size and strength of your calf muscles. Your legs will look and perform better, and it'll lower the risks of shin and knee injuries.

- Sit on the calf raise machine and place the front of your feet on the foot platform. Your heels should be extended out.
- Move your thighs under the pads and adjust to get a good fit.
- Release the safety bar by lifting the lever.
- Hold the handles for support and inhale as you allow the lever to descend in a controlled manner.
- Hold for a few seconds. Now exhale as you raise your heels and press the lever all the way up.
- Hold for a few seconds and repeat the movement as desired. Keep the repetitions slow and controlled.
- Secure the lever with the safety bar after completion.
- Repeat 3 sets of 8 reps.

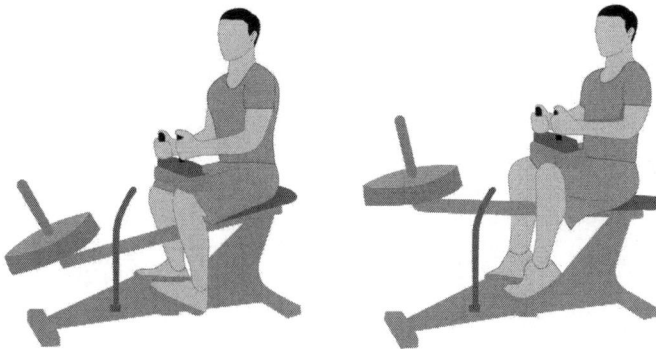

FIGURE 13-8: MACHINE SEATED CALF RAISE

BACK & SHOULDERS

#1 – Machine Cable Front Lat Pull-Downs

This exercise strengthens the latissimus dorsi muscle or lat. It's a broad muscle that extends under your armpits and spreads across and down your back.

- Sit comfortably on the seat with your feet flat on the floor.
- Ensure the bar is at a height where your outstretched arms can comfortably grasp it without standing up.
- Grasp the bar and pull down until it's level with your chin.
- Ensure your upper torso remains stationary and feet flat. Engage your abs as you pull.
- Stop at the bottom of the motion when your elbows can't move further down without moving backward.
- Squeeze your shoulder blades together and maintain square shoulders.
- Now return the bar slowly to the start position while controlling its gradual ascent. Don't let the weight plates crush.
- Perform 3 sets of 12 reps.

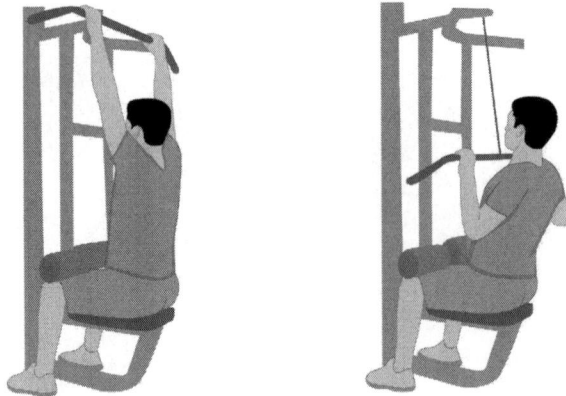

FIGURE 14-1: MACHINE CABLE FRONT LAT PULL-DOWNS

#2 – Body-Weight Chin-Ups

This exercise will help increase the strength and size of your upper back and arm muscles. It specifically targets the forearms, biceps, shoulders and lats.

- Start by grabbing the chin-up bar at shoulder width with an underhand grip. Your palms should be facing towards you.
- Hang from the bar in what's called a dead hang. Engage your core and tuck your chin with shoulder blades rotated upward.
- Initiate an upward movement by simultaneously pulling your shoulder blades down and your elbows towards your body.
- Continue until your shoulder bone reaches the chin-up bar.
- Hold for a few seconds. With a controlled motion, slowly lower yourself back down until your arms are straight.
- Repeat as required or until it gets difficult to pull yourself up.
- Aim for of 10 repetitions.

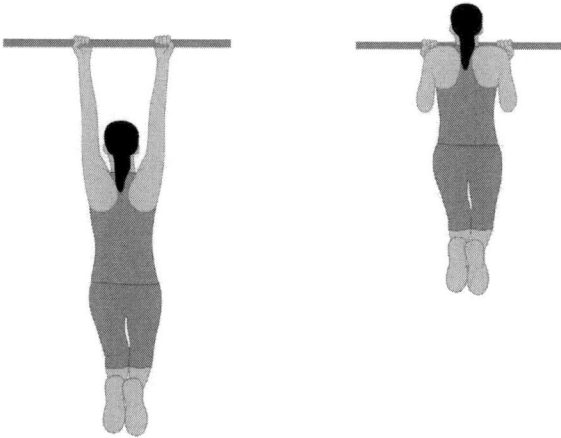

FIGURE 14-2: BODY WEIGHT CHIN-UPS

#3 – Standing Cable Pullover

This exercise helps build your lats' strength and size and targets the chest, shoulders, and middle back. It'll help you build upper-body mass and muscle definition.

- Attach a straight bar high up the cable station pulley.
- Grip the bar in an overhand position with your hands shoulder-width apart.
- Keep a 30-degree bend in your elbows.
- Maintain a solid stance with feet shoulder-width apart. They can be side by side or one foot slightly in front of the other.
- Pull the cable attachment down in a circular motion with your lower back naturally arched, chest puffed out and core tight.
- Keep your arms straight and focus on driving the resistance down with your elbows rather than your hands.
- When the bar reaches your thighs, pause for a few seconds.
- Slowly return the bar to the start position.
- Repeat 3 sets of 10-12 reps.

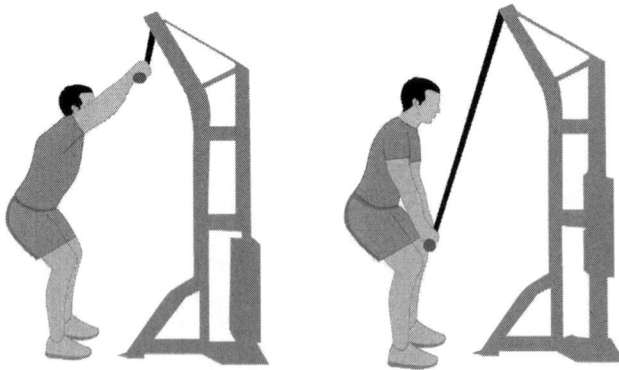

FIGURE 14-3: STANDING CABLE PULLOVER

#4 – Seated Low Cable Pulley Rows

This exercise will help strengthen and tone your lats and shoulder blade muscles. It also works on the trapezius (shoulders and upper back) and biceps brachii (upper arm).

- Start by adjusting the seat pad to ensure your shoulders are level with the machine handles.
- Sit upright on the platform with knees bent and feet firmly planted on the floor.
- Grasp the cable and move your shoulders back and down.
- Brace your core, exhale and pull the cable by bending your elbows.
- Keep your back straight, chest out, and squeeze your shoulder blades in as you row.
- Pause for a few seconds, inhale, and slowly extend your arms to return the cable forward.
- Repeat 3 sets of 12 reps.

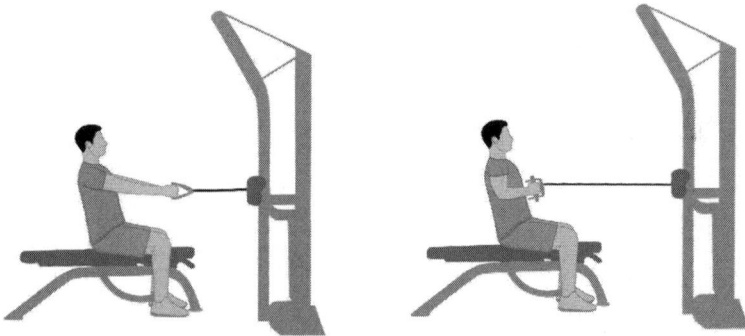

FIGURE 14-4: SEATED LOW CABLE PULLEY ROWS

#5 – Machine Shoulder Press

This exercise will help strengthen your shoulders and upper back. It targets the anterior deltoid (shoulder muscle) and works on the trapezius, triceps, and pectoral muscles.

- Adjust the seat to the correct height and sit with the handles at roughly shoulder height.
- Your back should stay straight and your core stiff or tight.
- Hold on to the handles and look straight ahead.
- Inhale and slowly press the handles up above your head.
- Ensure you don't lock out your elbows.
- Slowly your hands to about eye level to complete one rep.
- Note: you do not have to go all the way down.
- Repeat 3 sets of 10 reps.

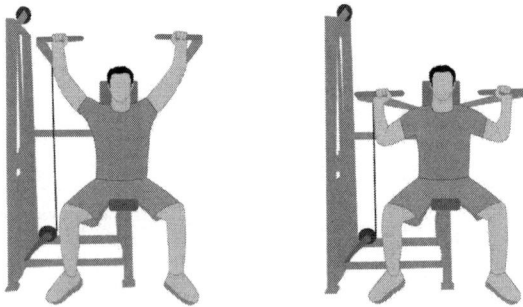

FIGURE 14-5: MACHINE SHOULDER PRESS

#6 – Rear Deltoid Machine

This exercise primarily focuses on strengthening your posterior deltoids. It also works on the trapezius, rhomboids, and other small muscles on your upper back.

- Sit and adjust the seat of the rear delt machine so your chest is pressed against the chest pad and handles are at shoulder level.
- Your back should be straight, and your feet planted firmly on the floor.
- Hold the handles in front of you and pull the machine's arms back with a slight bend in your elbows, like doing a reverse butterfly stroke.
- Pull back as far as you can without jerking your body.
- Stop when the handles reach your sides and slowly return to the starting position.
- Repeat 3 sets of 12 reps.
- TIP: Don't aim to lift heavy weights on this exercise. Focus on performing each rep mindfully with low weights.

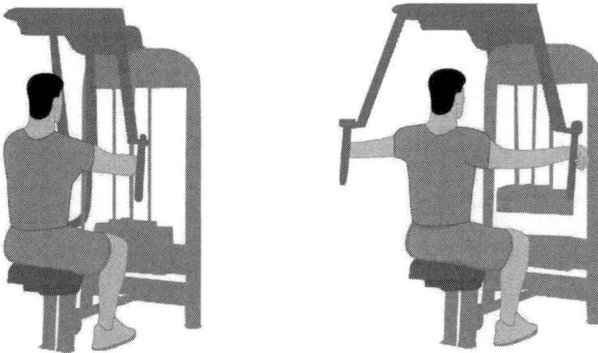

FIGURE 14-6: REAR DELTOID MACHINE

ARMS

#1 – Machine Cable Triceps Pushdown

This exercise increases the size and strength of your arms by working on the triceps brachii muscle found at the rear of your upper arm.

- Use the pin to set a low weight to start.
- Grasp the rope attachment or horizontal cable bar using an overhand grip while facing the triceps pushdown machine.
- Adjust the bar to about chest level.
- Position your feet slightly apart, tuck your elbows in at your sides and brace your abdominals.
- Inhale and push down until your elbows are fully extended but not yet in a locked, straight position.
- Keep your elbows close to your body.
- Ensure you don't bend forward and keep your back as straight as possible.
- Exhale and return to the start position in a controlled movement without crashing the weights.
- Repeat 3 sets of 10-12 reps.

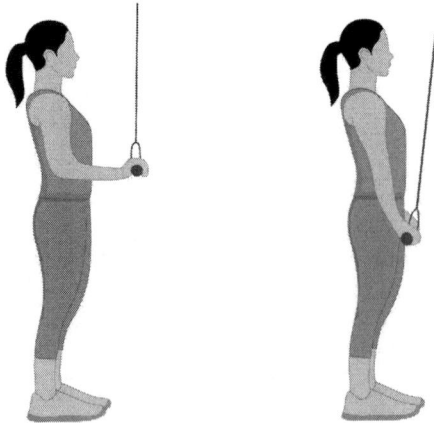

FIGURE 15-1: MACHINE CABLE TRICEP PUSHDOWNS

#2 – Bicep Curl Machine

This exercise is excellent for increasing the size and strength of your bicep muscles at the front of your upper arm and the muscles of your lower arm.

- Sit on the machine and place your arms on the inclined pad.
- Adjust the seat's height until the middle of your elbows is aligned with the rotation axis of the machine.
- Firmly grasp the handles and maintain a neutral wrist position.
- Stiffen your abdominal muscles and pull your shoulders back and down. Focus on keeping your back straight throughout the movements.
- Exhale and slowly curl the bar upwards towards your chest by bending your elbows.
- Continue bending upwards until your elbows can no longer bend.
- Pause for a moment and slowly return to the starting position by allowing your elbows to extend in a controlled movement.
- Repeat 3 sets of 10 reps.

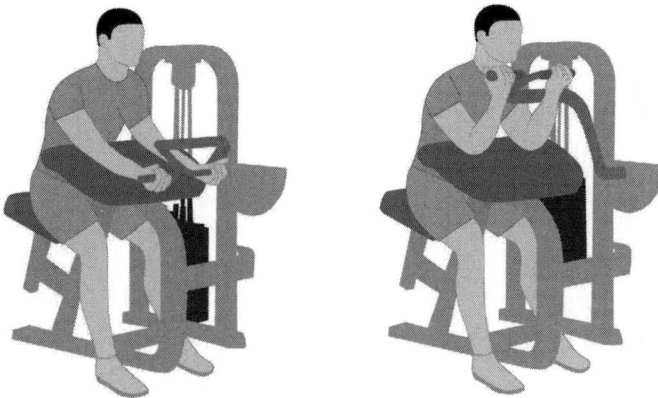

FIGURE 15-2: BICEP CURL MACHINE

Phew! Now that was quite a workout, wasn't it! Don't worry if the exercises seem complex to begin with. The more you try and practice, the easier it will become.

Let's move onto chapter eight, where we start our warm-up exercises and get ready for the workout routines.

8

WARMING UP FOR YOUR ROUTINE

In chapter five we showed you a few warm-up exercises. Here in chapter eight we're reviewing what we previously learned from that chapter, to help us prepare for the workout routines themselves. Warming up your muscles gets them to relax and become more supple. It also increases the overall flow of blood and oxygen to the muscles, ensuring that they are well-nourished throughout the exercise process.

DISCLAIMER

You should always consult with your physician or healthcare provider before changing your regular exercise program or trying new forms of exercise. You should not use the book's contents as a substitute for professional medical advice, treatment, or diagnosis.

The most important part of this process is realizing that you're kickstarting your body from sedentary into action, which has to be done slowly and steadily. Warm-ups should only be around five to ten minutes long. Start every strength training with this important step.

WARM-UP EXERCISES

Back Arch Stretch

Stand with your feet shoulder-width apart and gently lean back with your hands on your hips. Hold the position for a few seconds and gently return to your starting position. Repeat 3-4 times.

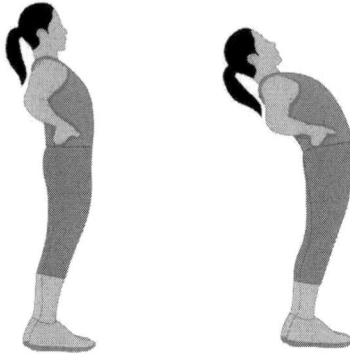

FIGURE 16-1: BACK ARCH STRETCH

Tricep Circles

Loosening and warming up your triceps is an important part of the process. You can do this with tricep circles. Do ten circles forward, then rotate the opposite direction doing another ten.

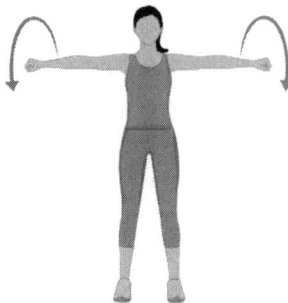

FIGURE 16-2: TRICEP CIRCLES

Wall Pushups

Instead of doing a regular push-up, we will do wall push-ups until you have built enough strength to try doing push-ups the traditional way (on the ground). Wall push-ups warm up your arms, shoulders, and chest. Do ten to fifteen to warm up.

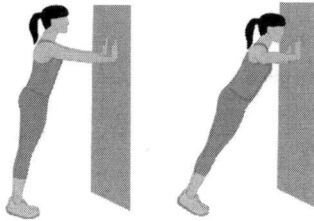

FIGURE 16-3: WALL PUSHUPS

Walk/Run on the Spot

Of course, you need to get your heart rate slightly up so that it's ready for your workout. You can do this by running or walking fast on the spot for a few minutes.

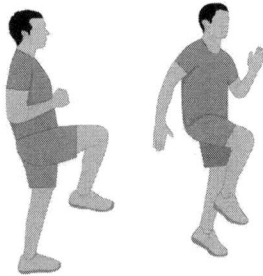

FIGURE 16-4: WALK/JOG ON THE SPOT

EXTRA ITEMS TO HAVE HANDY

***Reminder**: Make sure that you have these items before you get started with your workout routine.

Exercise mat (the thicker, the better) if you don't have a mat for now, a very thick folded towel can be a good substitute.

Towel (to dry up any sweat, yes, you're going to sweat)

Water bottle (staying hydrated between exercises is essential) take small sips of water when you can throughout your workout. Don't gulp a lot, as it will just make you feel uncomfortable.

If you're exercising outside, make sure that you have sunscreen or a hat to protect you from the sun.

Good pair of exercise shoes, gym floor shoes or running shoes will suffice. Don't attempt to do exercise in your regular shoes as they don't provide sufficient grip or support.

Suitable exercise clothes. Choose clothes that are fitted without being too tight. If your clothing is too loose and baggy, it will just get in the way and make you feel hot. A tee-shirt or vest and sweatpants or shorts (or yoga tights) are suitable.

9

THE 20-MINUTE WORKOUT

OVERVIEW OF THE WORKOUT

Here's an entry level full-body workout that you can do at home. We know that life can get a little busy, and a 20-minute workout (three times per week) will be the perfect way for you to reclaim your health. This routine does not require equipment and can be done using little floor space. It effectively targets all major muscle groups; chest, legs, shoulders, arms, back, and core. Make sure to take a 1-2 minute break between sets as you move through each exercise.

THE ROUTINE AT A GLANCE

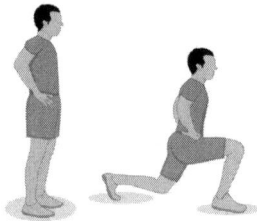

1. BASIC LUNGES: 2 SETS OF 10 REPS - EACH SIDE

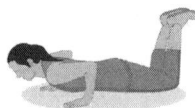

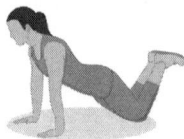

2. MODIFIED PUSH-UPS: 3 SETS OF 10 REPS

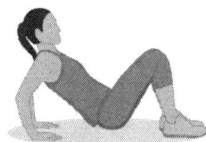

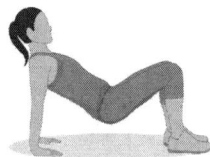

3. GROUND TRICEP DIPS: 3 SETS OF 10 REPS

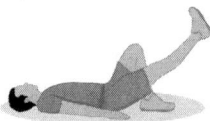

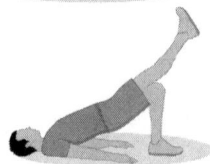

4. HAMSTRING BRIDGE: 2 SETS OF 10 REPS - EACH SIDE

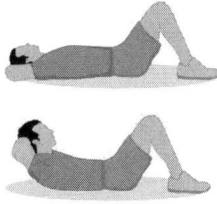

5. BASIC AB CRUNCHES: 2 SETS OF 20 REPS

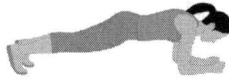

6. PLANKS: 3 SETS OF 30-SECOND HOLDS

COOL DOWN & FOLLOW-UP

A cool down period for a 20-minute workout should last at least five minutes, and can involve walking and doing some stretching. This is important for the following reasons: it regulates blood flow and promotes a gradual recovery of heart rate and blood pressure. If this is the first routine you've completed in a while, congratulations, you're on your way. Keep going. Start a habit. Eventually you'll want to get this routine up to 3 times per week. It will get easier with every passing week.

---

*Your fitness level.
If you find that you need more of a challenge, no worries, let's move you on! The next chapter shows a 40-minute routine that involves equipment. Here's where we start implementing some additional tools. So roll out your dumbbells, stability ball and stretching bands.

10

THE 40-MINUTE WORKOUT

OVERVIEW OF THE WORKOUT

The 40-minute full-body workout can be done either at home (if you have basic equipment) or at a gym. Aim for 3 sessions per week. It's here where you'll build a solid workout plan and make it part of your weekly activities. All major muscle groups are targeted; legs, chest, shoulders, back, arms and core. The results will increase your muscle strength and boost your energy levels. Remember to warm up prior to the workout and cool-down just after finishing.

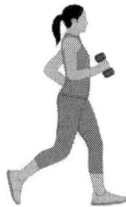

LET'S GET STARTED!

THE ROUTINE AT A GLANCE

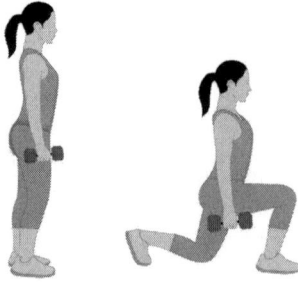

1. WEIGHTED LUNGES: 2 SETS OF 10 REPS - EACH SIDE

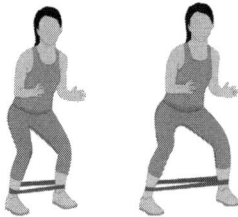

2. RESISTANCE LATERAL WALK: 2 SETS OF 10 REPS

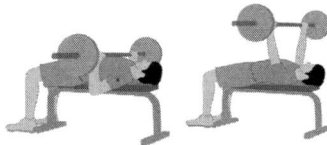

3. BARBELL BENCH PRESS: 3 SETS OF 10 REPS

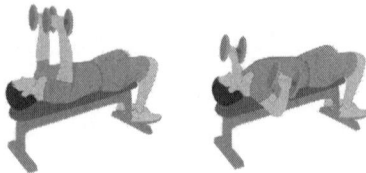

4. DUMBBELL BENCH FLYES: 3 SETS OF 10 REPS

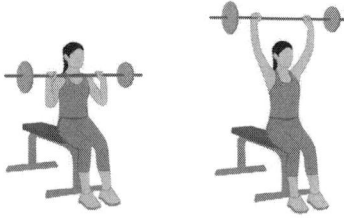

5. BARBELL SEATED SHOULDER PRESS: 3 SETS OF 8 REPS

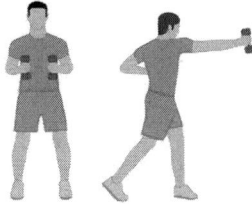

6. BOXING WITH HAND WEIGHTS: 30 ALTERNATING PUNCHES

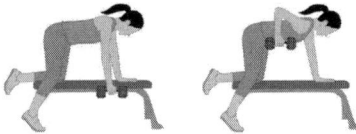

7. DUMBBELL ROWS: 2 SETS OF 10 REPS - EACH SIDE

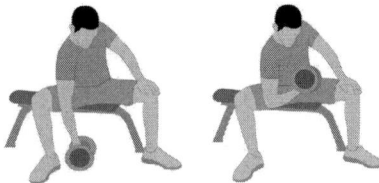

8. DUMBBELL CURL: 2 SETS OF 10 REPS - EACH SIDE

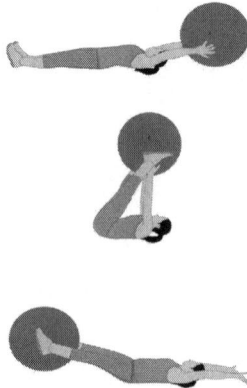

9. STABILITY BALL HANDS-TO-FEET: 2 SETS OF 8 REPS

COOL DOWN & FOLLOW-UP

A cool down period for a 40-minute workout should last at least ten minutes, and can involve walking or jogging on the spot, and doing some stretching. This is important for the following reasons: it regulates blood flow and promotes a gradual recovery of heart rate and blood pressure. This is a full-body workout routine that you'll want to keep up with at least 3 times per week. Develop the habit and it will get easier with every passing week.

*Your fitness level.
It's important to know where your current fitness level is at so you can start out with the proper weights. Dumbbells and barbells are not a "one-size-fits-all". You don't want a weight that is too light or too heavy. The proper weight is the one that makes you struggle to get the last few reps in. Listen to your body and make sure you test it through a trial and error process.

11

THE 60-MINUTE WORKOUT

OVERVIEW OF THE WORKOUT

This 60-minute full-body workout is one you'll do at the gym. A full-body workout means that you are exercising all the muscle groups in one single workout. It combines the upper body, the lower body, and the core all in one training session. Schedule this workout every second day. Many fitness instructors advise to do a cardio session right after the strength training routine to avoid fatiguing the muscles prior to the workout. It's important to start with ten minutes of pre-workout warm-up, as we covered in chapter eight. Add in jumping jacks, skipping, and butt kicks to your warm-up.

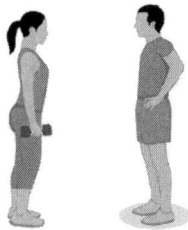

LET'S GET STARTED!

THE ROUTINE AT A GLANCE

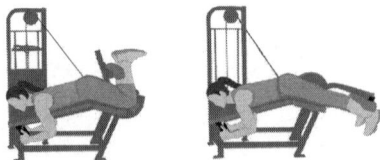

1. MACHINE LYING LEG CURL: 3 SETS OF 10 REPS

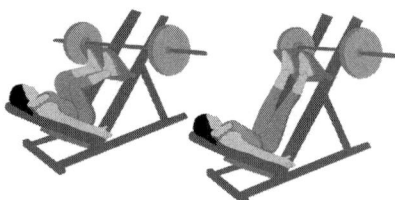

2. MACHINE INCLINE LEG PRESS: 3 SETS OF 8 REPS

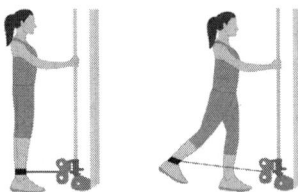

3. CABLE HIP EXTENSIONS: 2 SETS OF 10 REPS - EACH SIDE

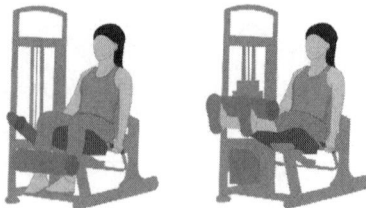

4. MACHINE SEATED LEG EXTENSIONS: 3 SETS OF 10 REPS

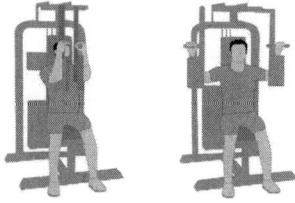

5. PEC DECK MACHINE: 4 SETS OF 8 REPS

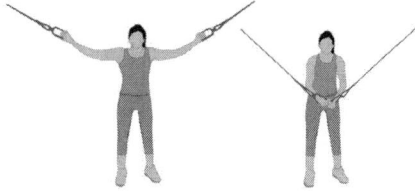

6. CABLE CROSSOVER: 3 SETS OF 10 REPS

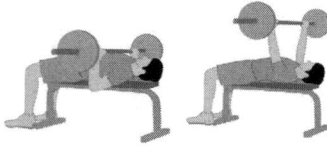

7. BARBELL BENCH PRESS: 3 SETS OF 10 REPS

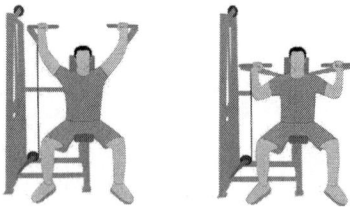

8. MACHINE SHOULDER PRESS: 3 SETS OF 10 REPS

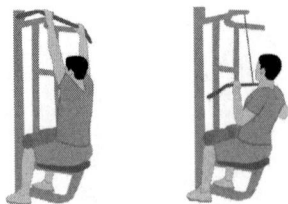

9. MACHINE CABLE LAT PULL-DOWNS: 3 SETS OF 12 REPS

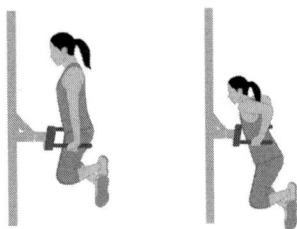

10. BODY WEIGHT DIPS: 2 SETS OF 10 REPS

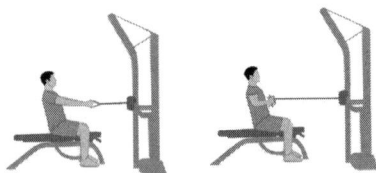

11. SEATED CABLE PULLEY ROWS: 3 SETS OF 10 REPS

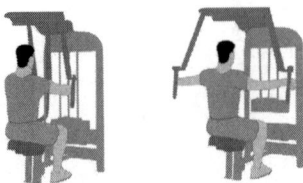

12. REAR DELTOID MACHINE: 3 SETS OF 8 REPS

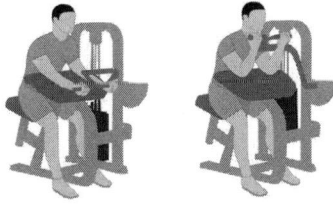

13. BICEP CURL MACHINE: 3 SETS OF 10 REPS

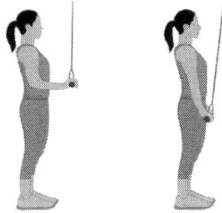

14. CABLE TRICEP PUSHDOWNS: 3 SETS OF 12 REPS

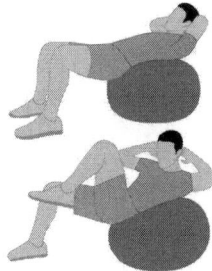

15. STABILITY BICYCLE CRUNCH: 15 REPS EACH SIDE

COOL DOWN & FOLLOW-UP

Once you're finished your workout routine, take a few minutes to cool down with lower-intensity movement. A cool-down period for a 90-minute workout routine should last ten minutes This will regulate your blood flow and promotes a gradual recovery of heart rate and blood pressure. Make sure to stretch your muscles and hold each stretch for ten seconds. A proper cool-down period can involve walking or jogging (can be jogging on the spot) and doing some basic stretching of most major muscles.

---

*Your fitness level.

Phew! Now that's a great workout, isn't it! Don't worry if the exercises seem complex to begin with. The more you try and practice, the easier it will become. Let's move onto chapter 12 where you'll learn tips and advice for maintaining your long-term health.

12

STAYING FIT & HEALTHY, LONG TERM

Now that you have learned all about the health benefits of strength training and gone through a range of exercises from the most basic to the more complex involving gym equipment, you feel you're ready and rearing to go.

The only problem is that often newfound motivation and enthusiasm dwindle, and soon you're back to old ways. You might find yourself lazing in bed an hour longer instead of doing your exercises. You may catch the bus or find yourself driving to the store when it's genuinely close enough to walk. You might even find yourself uttering the dreaded words, "not today, I'm too tired".

One way to safeguard yourself from slipping into old ways and neglecting your health and fitness is to create a healthy and strong foundation. While you probably won't change your life and behaviors overnight, you can work on actively making strength training and healthy choices a habit instead of a chore. The first step is to develop healthy habits.

HOW TO DEVELOP HEALTHY HABITS

The thing about habits is that we do them without thinking. For example, brushing our teeth is a habit; eating is a habit; how you react to people is a habit. These are things you do automatically. With this in mind, it's reasonable to think that you need to make it a habit if you want to keep up with your strength training long-term. Being consistent and forcing yourself to practice even when you don't want to is a good step in the right direction. Sure, it sounds uncomfortable to "force" yourself to do anything, but it's really just a short-term struggle you will have with your mind. As soon as your mind (remember we spoke about developing the right mindset) is on board, a habit can form. And then you're onto a good thing. Then strength training will just be part of your day, like eating and breathing.

It took us about six weeks to turn our curiosity about exercise into a habit. Actually, for us, it's become more of a full-blown addiction! For us, aging isn't about "getting old." Healthy aging, in our opinion, is about staying physically active, finding new things to enjoy, and connecting with family and friends. For many people, growing older brings fear and anxiety that stem from misconceptions. The reality is that you are more potent and resilient than you realize. With the right approach, you can maintain your emotional and physical health; and thrive, whatever the circumstances or your age. To help you along the way, we're going to share a few tips for developing healthy habits with you. See them below.

1. The Time to Make Healthy Food Choices is Now!

In our 50s, we've seen some other 50+ers make some questionable food choices along the way. We've heard every excuse in the book, from "We're old enough to eat what we want now" to "Who do I need to look good for anyway?" In the end, these are just excuses. Eating healthy can be tough. It almost seems like we revert to the convenient meals we wanted in our teens. As Jerry Rice says, "Do today what other people won't so that tomorrow you do what they can't."

Making healthy food choices now will do great things for your future health. And it's not about limiting yourself to bland meals or eating purely for good looks. What you eat can impact your body's ability to cope and, of course, either strengthen or weaken you to diseases.

First and foremost, we don't expect you to eat a diet as sparse as a runway model. Instead, we recommend adopting a *healthier* approach. That doesn't mean skipping on burger night with your friends. Instead, go to burger night but consider a side salad instead of fries and skip on the bun for a bun-less burger option! If you eat cereal in the morning, look for sugar-free varieties and add a few pieces of fruit to add in. Let's talk about vitamins and minerals. When you're on the horizon of 50, your bones weaken, and your muscle mass declines. Now is a good time to increase your intake of calcium and vitamin D. The big 5-0 is also a time when lethargy kicks in and energy levels do a disappearing act. This can be a result of vitamin B12 deficiency. While you should aim to get most of your nutrition from your food, taking a decent multivitamin isn't a bad idea.

2. Reduce Caffeine and Sugar

We're probably going to be boo'd right out of the 50+ club with this one, but caffeine and sugar don't really serve you well. In fact, they take away from you. Too much caffeine robs you of your own personal energy, and soon, you become reliant on it. As you get older, it's also a bit of a sleep deterrent. At times, we've had our share of too much coffee, and we noticed just how restless sleep can be as a result. *"But coffee smells so good in the morning!"* Yes, but be aware that it can rob you of your sleep, and can also increase anxiety and lead to irregular heartbeats. It can be an issue when you have a heart condition. Sugary drinks and sodas can also be tempting. However, they contain high amounts of sugar that lead to health issues like obesity. Sugar can also significantly increase inflammation and irritation in the body, which is bad news for people with arthritis.

3. Schedule Workouts

After 50 you begin experiencing signs of aging that include loss of muscle mass, lower bone density, general weakness, slouching, and low metabolic rate. It certainly sounds like something you have to look forward to, doesn't it! We've already discussed the many exercises you can do to ensure that you reverse these signs of aging and live a more flexible, agile life – it's all about improved quality of life in the end.

The hard part isn't knowing what to do; it's sticking to it. Unfortunately, it's easy to lose interest or get busy with other things. You know the whole *"I will workout tomorrow"* excuse! We know how it goes because we were once in the very same predicament. The best way to overcome this problem is to develop a workout schedule and actually block off time in your diary. If you know that you exercise from 7 am to 7.45 am every Monday, Wednesday, and Friday, it will be easier for you to form a habit than if you just leave it up in the air. To ensure that you stick it out, invite someone to join you. Your partner, child, or friend will help you stick to your plans.

Another way of ensuring that your workout times become a habit is to choose the same time to work out every time and to ensure that it's at a time where other commitments are unlikely to crop up and interfere. If you find that an hour before bed is the only time that can happen, then so be it! We find that first thing in the morning is the best time for us. It gives us a burst of energy and endorphins for the day, and once it's out the way, we have time to do all the things we want to do that day. Freedom!

4. Make Active Hobbies Your Thing

Now that you're heading past 50 and toward the golden years, you might have time for hobbies. And hobbies are great at this stage of life. Hobbies help individuals shape their personality, act as inspiration, energize lifestyle, and connect with like-minded people. Engaging in a hobby will also provide mental health benefits and fill you with a sense of achievement. Avoid only engaging in hobbies that are sedentary. Be strategic about your hobby choices, as you can use them to maintain an active lifestyle.

Some obvious active hobbies include:

· Joining niegborhood runs

· Playing tennis

· Lawn bowling

· Learning Tai Chi

· Joining a walking group

· Walking the dog

· Playing catch with the grandkids

· Doing weekly gardening

· Hiking

· Playing golf

These are just a few ideas. Active hobbies help to tone, shape, and strengthen muscles, reduce weight, and increase energy levels. They are also great for cardiovascular health.

5. Find a Fitness Buddy

For us, we're lucky in that we have each other. We hold each other accountable for being fit and strong, and the fact that we have each other keeps us motivated, dedicated, and hardworking.

If you have a partner who will join you, great! If you don't - perhaps it's time to find someone who will join you with your workouts. Most 50+ers report that an active fitness buddy helps them achieve their fitness goals and stay committed to the process. Ask a friend or family member to join you, or if you're struggling to find someone, see if another 50+er in your community might be interested in getting active. It's worth it!

6. Track Your Progress

We strongly recommend that you start tracking your progress from day one. Make a list of what you want to achieve from your strength training efforts. Your list might look like this:

· Weight loss

· Getting stronger

· Relieve aches and pains

· Feel more energetic

· Competitive in sports

Then make a list of your current measurements. Note down your height, weight, measurements over your stomach, waist, legs, and arms. Record your clothing size and take a before picture so you can compare it with an after picture in a few weeks. When you start working out, set goals for yourself. Note how heavy your first weights are or how many reps you can achieve before getting tired. If you see that you can only manage using a 3-pound dumbbell this week, try to work your way up to using a 5-pound dumbbell in a fortnight. Each week, make a new note of how you have improved. As you see your progress climbing, you will undoubtedly feel motivated to push harder and achieve more. Seeing a visual representation of your progress is also good for your mental health. Achieving goals isn't a passive thing! As Jerry Dunn once said, "Don't limit challenges; instead, challenge your limits!" To reach your fitness goals, write them down on paper, create a strategic plan for achieving them (following the exercise advice in this book), acknowledge possible hurdles, make the required sacrifices, talk to others about the challenges, and act every single day on achieving that goal.

THE IMPORTANCE OF REST & RELAXATION

Did you know that the human body has an adverse to a lack of sleep and rest? If you don't get enough sleep and rest, it can obliterate your sex drive and weaken your overall immunity. It can also lead to weight gain and cognitive issues. And just when you think it can't get any worse, you can also increase your risk of getting diabetes or cancer. As a result, we always recommend resting between exercises and also taking days off from your workouts to get proper rest and repair. This forms part of your body's maintenance plan – which is very important when you're 50+! Let's look at a few aspects of healthy rest and relaxation.

1. Rest between sets of exercises

When following our exercise routines, you will notice that we recommend a minute or two rest between sets. When you rest between sets, your body energy system recuperates after exhausting the supplies, powering you up for a fresh set of bicep curls or another sprint. Without rest, you're working with tired muscles. When working out with tired muscles, you compromise good form, which can lead to injury.

2. Take days off and get enough sleep

Although taking breaks between sets is critical, the rest that happens between your workouts is even more important. This is because your body needs 48 - 72 hours of rest to repair muscles and recuperate fully after workouts. Of course, this all depends on the overall intensity of the workouts you are doing. For example, if you are only doing ten bicep curls a day, you don't really need rest days in between.

When it comes to strength training, we recommend resting for one day between workouts. Strength training every second day is a great way to ensure your muscles recover and that you have enough energy to put all of your strength into your next workout.

Many people overlook sleep, though it's critical in the process of recovery. Sleeping enables you to repair internally, including hormone levels and torn muscle tissues. Sleep allows your body to synthesize proteins at a higher rate too, which promotes muscle gain. Aim to get around seven hours of sleep per night.

KNOW YOUR WHY

We all have our reasons for wanting to get fit and active again, and that's what you should hold onto. Knowing what inspired interest in getting active again will help you realize your "why." In our opinion, there are many reasons why 50+ers should want to do strength training. Here's a look at some of them.

1. Helps combat chronic diseases and illnesses

Strength training improves the functioning of the digestive system and immune response, increases bone density, lowers blood pressure, and minimizes the risk of diseases such as obesity, diabetes, and Alzheimer's disease.

2. Increases confidence

50+ is a challenging time. It's a time of change, and often, those changes leave us feeling uncomfortable and awkward. It can be a real confidence knock. Our children move out of the nest, friends pass away, and retirement comes looking for us. Yikes. Strength training provides a burst of endorphins and leads to your looking and feeling great. It's hard not to feel confident when you feel this way.

3. Reduces inflammation

Low-grade inflammation leads to chronic conditions that lead to disability, mainly in older people. Regular exercise reduces pain and inflammation in the body.

4. Enhances flexibility, balance, and mobility

Through regular exercise, you attain better flexibility, posture, and strength. All these are vital for better coordination and balance.

STAYING MOTIVATED

Motivation is probably one of the most elusive things in the 50+ world. One moment you're motivated to do something, and the next, you're daydreaming of lazing on the sofa doing nothing. Getting older means that motivation escapes you from time to time, but it doesn't have to be a long-term thing. As we already mentioned, it's all about developing a habit. Motivation is all about establishing long-lasting behavior change. To avoid getting sidetracked, especially if you're prone to losing interest in new activities, follow these tips to help stay motivated.

1. Concentrate on the short-term goals

If you're overly focused on your main goal, you're going to feel despondent early on in the process. If you want to shed loads of weight and go down three jeans sizes, you can't keep thinking of that. Set a shorter small goal that you can achieve on the way. For instance, going down just one jeans size to start with is an excellent short-term goal. For us, targeting mood and energy level enhancement was a great short-term goal.

2. Reward yourself for the small achievements

Each time you complete a small milestone, reward yourself. It can be a simple activity like remembering to go for a walk or managing to do a few extra reps in your strength training workout. Your rewards can include a hot bath, a favorite beverage, or something you thoroughly enjoy! The human brain (and body) loves rewards, so this is a great strategy if you're trying to make strength training a habit!

3. Cultivate a supportive environment

Make plans to exercise with a loved one as they can encourage and nudge you on. A supportive environment consisting of friends and family is important when trying to get fit and healthy again. When you're trying something new, like going for Sunday morning walks, for instance, encouraging your support system to join you is a great idea. Not only will you feel supported, but you will get to spend a bit of quality time with your loved ones. Another way to gather support and stay motivated as a result is to join an online community where other 50+ers are active and getting in shape. Simply connecting with like-minded people or sharing your small successes along the way will do wonders for your mindset and motivation too.

5. Have an alternative plan

Since life is not a straight line, there are bound to be moments when unpredictable events happen or potential barriers arise. It's smart to have a decent backup plan in place to mitigate these moments. For instance, have a few items of equipment (dumbbells, balance ball, stretch band) at home so you can still do a workout if it rains and you have to cancel your walk/run.

Prioritizing Your Mental Health

Welcome to 50! Please select a mental health condition and spend the rest of your life dealing with it. Okay, that sounds like a pretty bleak announcement, but it's true. Most people suffer some form of mental health problem at some stage in their lives, and the reality is that we're more prone to mental health concerns as we get older. Some put it down to living a long life and knowing all that we do! Others realize that it's loss, physical pain, illness, and often the act of neglecting oneself that can lead to a mental downturn. Some of the common mental health problems that plague 50+ers include the following:

1. Anxiety
2. Memory problems
3. Severe cognitive impairment
4. Depression
5. Cognitive decline
6. Mood disorders
7. Persistent stress
8. Addiction

You probably already know that we're going to say the number one of overcoming and reducing the symptoms of mental health issues is exercise. And we are going to say that because it's true! Exercise reduces anxiety and depression and improves mood, cognitive function, and self-esteem.

Of course, we also promote mental health through having a reliable and supportive social network. If you don't have a lot of family and friends to rely on, consider joining a community exercise class so that you can meet other 50+ers with the same health priorities as you. If you have some relatives and friends who live far away, get into the habit of calling them and checking in – sometimes social connection, even over the telephone, is enough for a mental and emotional boost.

Lastly, mental health also relies on mental sharpness, and it's one of the things we wanted to come through quite strongly in this book. Learning new things and engaging your mind is essential for cognitive function and mental sharpness.

Simply focusing on the exercises in this book will go a long way toward fully engaging your mental capacity.

Read as much as you can, learn new things as much as you can and keep engaging with puzzles, hobbies, activities, and outings. The more active you keep your body *and* mind, the healthier you will be physically and mentally.

Being mentally healthy means you're happy, at peace, and satisfied with life. This translates to a meaningful existence filled with a sense of purpose and peace. In addition, you're better able to cope with life's challenges as you're confident with elevated self-esteem and optimism. And if strength training is the first step you take towards experiencing and enjoying all of this, why not!

Now, you're almost ready to take all your strength training knowledge and put it to good use. Before you go, turn over to the final page for a few last words from the authors.

OUR FINAL WORD

We've taken quite the journey together, haven't we? At first, we merely approached the topic of strength training and how it can benefit your life. Then, we dove right in and got you excited about it. We undoubtedly had you nodding along in agreement as we described the various aches, pains, and challenges that face most 50+ club members. But then, just when you were ready to accept your fate of aches, pains, and inflexibility, receive your old-age certificate, and settle in for the next trying phase of life, we gave you a truth bomb! Old age is all in your head.

It can be in your body too, but that's only if you neglect your body. Think of your body like a property you invest in. If your children had their eye on a beautiful house to invest in, what type of advice would you give them, over above the typical money advice? You'd probably tell them that the cost of the house is not the only cost they will pay. You will probably draw their attention to how the neighborhood (environment) will change over the years, and all the time and effort they *must* put in to care for and maintain their property. If they don't, what will happen? The house will crack, fade, and weaken. It will start to fall apart, the roof will leak, and dampness will settle in. Ultimately, the house will lose its value. On the contrary, being willing to invest the time and energy for ongoing maintenance over the years will ensure that the house remains valuable, prime, and in excellent condition. As a result, it won't become a financial burden or a health hazard to your children and grandchildren. This advice is something you can apply to your own life. Think of your body as your home – it's your property. In fact, it's your greatest investment. It didn't cost you a cent, but it could cost you your life (and life enjoyment) if you don't put time and effort into maintaining it. That's enough property analogies for now.

Now is the time to take the next step: getting active. You have all the strength training advice you need to get started and a plethora of exercises to try at home without equipment, with equipment, and even at the gym. There are no more excuses – you're fully equipped. Before you start with your first strength training exercises (we know you're dying to get started), we'd love to extend a heartfelt gratitude to you. Thank you for purchasing our book and trusting us to guide you on your strength training journey. If you enjoyed what you've learned here, please reach out with an honest review.

Best of luck!

Alicia & Lee

If you enjoyed this book, please leave us a review.
We'd love to hear from you. Thank you!

SCAN ME

Printed in Great Britain
by Amazon